Caring
for the
Vascular Patient

For Churchill Livingstone:

Commissioning Editor: Ellen Green
Project Manager: Valerie Burgess
Project Development Editor: Mairi McCubbin
Design Direction: Judith Wright
Medical Illustrator: Robert Britton
Diagrammatic illustrations: Alan Palfreyman
Copy-editor: Colin Nicholls
PTU operator: Gerard Heyburn
Indexer: Liza Weinkove
Sales promotion executive: Hilary Brown

Caring
for the
Vascular Patient

Lynda M. Herbert RGN
Vascular Nurse Practitioner
Good Hope Hospital NHS Trust
Sutton Coldfield, UK

Foreword by

Ian S. Paterson MD FRCS
Royal College of Surgeons Hunterian Professor of Surgery 1996–1997;
Consultant Vascular Surgeon, Good Hope NHS Trust, Sutton Coldfield;
Honorary Senior Lecturer, University of Birmingham, Birmingham, UK

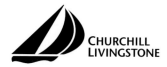

CHURCHILL
LIVINGSTONE

NEW YORK EDINBURGH LONDON MADRID MELBOURNE SAN FRANCISCO AND TOKYO 1997

CHURCHILL LIVINGSTONE
Medical Division of Pearson Professional Limited

Distributed in the United States of America by Churchill Livingstone Inc., 650 Avenue of the Americas, New York, N.Y. 10011, and by associated companies, branches and representatives throughout the world.

First published 1997

ISBN 0 443 05423 1

British Library of Cataloguing in Publication Data
A catalogue record for this book is available from the British Library.

Library of Congress Cataloging in Publication Data
A catalog record for this book is available from the Library of Congress.

Medical knowledge is constantly changing. As new information becomes available, changes in treatment, procedures, equipment and the use of drugs become necessary. The editors / authors / contributors and publishers have, as far as it is possible, taken care to ensure that the information given in this text is accurate and up to date. However, readers are strongly advised to confirm that the information, especially with regard to drug usage, complies with current legislation and standards of practice.

The
publisher's
policy is to use
paper manufactured
from sustainable forests

Produced by Longman Singapore Publishers Pte Ltd
Printed in Singapore

Contents

Foreword

I am delighted to be asked to provide the foreword for what I think is an important work in the development of specialist vascular nursing in this country. In the United Kingdom, the majority of peripheral vascular surgery is carried out in District General Hospitals, and the management of patients with arterial venous problems represents an increasing commitment for general surgical wards and their nursing staff. Perhaps more than in any other surgical speciality, the pace of development in vascular surgery, particularly with regard to more complex reconstruction and endovascular techniques, has increased. These, together with a better understanding of the disease processes at the microvascular level, have meant that more and more can be done for an increasing number of patients with vascular disease. It is often difficult for specialists in the field to keep abreast of new developments and for these to be effectively communicated to primary care physicians and the nurses who are caring for the patients in the ward and the community. This book will prove invaluable in both of these spheres to increase knowledge and to help improve informed patient care.

This book represents not only a great deal of time, effort and dedication on the part of the author but is also the culmination of three years' hard work to fund and establish the unique post of vascular nurse practitioner. The role itself has expanded and encompasses many areas described in the chapters of this book. For the sake of the development of vascular surgical services throughout the country I hope that nurses elsewhere will not only feel more competent in dealing with their vascular patients, but will also be enthusiastic enough about this new type of post to want to become involved.

I. S. Paterson
Sutton Coldfield

Acknowledgements

The author acknowledges with gratitude the support received from Tim Muscroft, Consultant Surgeon, who kindly proofread the manuscript in great depth. Gratitude is also extended to the following people for their support and provision of resources that have contributed to the quality of this book: Michael Crowson, FRCS; Ian Paterson, MD, FRCS; Edward Millar, FRCR; Adrian Parnell, MRCP, FRCR; Paula Ghanah, FRCS; Angela Reynolds, BA, RGN, CertEd; Gwyn Giles (Librarian), Good Hope Hospital Trust, Sutton Coldfield; Christine Moffatt, RGN, DDN; Madeleine Flanagan, BSc, RGN, ONC, DipN, RNT, CertN.

I should also like to thank my parents, Norman and Irene Baybutt, my husband, Trefor Herbert, MA, MRCGP, and my children, Emma, Matthew, Simon and David, for their support, encouragement and practical help.

Acknowledgement is also due to the following organizations: Smith and Nephew; Convatec; Beiersdorf; Huntleight Health Care; Medi UK; Vessa Ltd; Impra UK; 3M Health Care.

Finally, recognition and thanks are extended to the patients who have shared with the author their experiences, and kindly permitted their photographs to be used to illustrate this text.

Introduction

Amputation is the oldest form of operation, yet only recently, with the advent of modern technology, has the profile of *vascular surgery* risen greatly. Surgeons are now in a position to perform procedures and operations for which they previously did not have the resources, and ischaemic patients are able to reap the benefits of microsurgical techniques.

Vascular surgical patients who have undergone major surgery, and who at one time spent a considerable time in intensive care, are now transferred back to the ward more quickly and are discharged sooner into the community. *Nurses have a responsibility to be able to adequately care for these patients, basing their practice on sound research-based knowledge.*

From the evaluation of an audit performed by the author, it became evident that patients and practitioners would benefit from increased information to help them make *informed choices*. If practitioners have access to sound information, they are in a better position to help patients make informed choices, in line with the *Patients' Charter*.

The aim of this book is to provide a ready reference for those interested in the field of peripheral vascular disease. The book is not intended to be prescriptive but permissive, and offers information that will assist in the gathering of *research-based information*, so aiding practitioners to acquire a compassionate understanding of the *specific needs of patients in vascular surgery*. Recognition is given to the fact that there will be regional differences in practice regarding individual situations.

The acquisition of sound knowledge is essential to the *Scope of Professional Practice*. All practitioners are well aware that *'being accountable for one's own Practice'* is a responsibility they cannot afford to take lightly.

It is hoped that this book will be useful to practitioners at all levels, from the student working towards a diploma or degree to the qualified practitioner in either the primary or the secondary area of care, who is looking to update his or her practice and level of knowledge in line with *Post-Registration Education and Practice (PREP)*. The author has followed the *principle of applying knowledge to practice*, with the aim of allowing the practitioner to *assess* fully the needs of vascular patients, *plan* their care appropriately, *implement* care and adequately *evaluate* the outcomes.

Shared knowledge of this patient group's needs between the primary and secondary sectors will help to provide a *'seamless service'*.

During the course of their treatment, patients will come into contact with professionals from many disciplines. It is therefore hoped that the information contained herein will be useful to all members of the multidisciplinary team, encouraging an understanding of the *holistic management* these patients require.

The book addresses a wide range of subject-matter related to the vascular field, including *clinical guidelines* for the care of each vascular patient group and examples of care using a *nursing model* for each group. Effective management of *pain and wounds* is also addressed.

It is anticipated that early *health promotion* can effectively reduce the incidence of vascular disease. Reference is therefore made to issues surrounding this, as the role of any practitioner is to help prevent disease where possible through the counselling of patients, both young and old.

It is hoped that the information provided will promote the *delivery of high standards of care* which are *measurable* within the *audit cycle* and which are seen to be of great benefit to patients, to their relatives and to the service in general.

For practitioners, it is as important to consider the *ethics of practice* as it is the implementation of care. This is borne in mind in the presentation of the text.

Each chapter is intended to be self-contained in that it can be read in isolation by the practitioner who wishes to revise the nursing management of a particular procedure. For this reason a degree of repetition in different chapters is inevitable.

Throughout the text, the *highlighting* of *key terminology* will be presented by *italics* and *signposting*, so enabling the practitioner readily to extract information. It is hoped that the *cross-referencing* and *further reading lists* will make this book a valuable resource.

Background

SECTION

1

Anatomy and physiology of the vascular system

This chapter seeks to give an overview of the structure and function of the circulatory system and related structures. It investigates the constituents of blood, including the blood gases. Finally the physiology of wound healing is examined.

THE ARTERIAL SYSTEM

The arterial system, as seen in Figure 1.1, is responsible for ensuring that a blood supply, rich in nutrients, is able to reach the peripheral vascular beds.

The structure of arteries

The walls of the *arteries* comprise three distinct layers, the *intima*, the *media* and the *adventitia* (Fig. 1.2).

The *intima* of the arteries is a *single layer* of pavement-like *endothelial cells* on a layer of connective tissue, with a layer of elastic membrane to separate it from the medial layer. As endothelial cells are smooth, they reduce the risk of blood clotting as it passes over the correct surface for the lumen of a vessel.

The *media* is predominantly composed of smooth (non-striated) muscle. *Arteries* tend to be *thicker* than veins as their medial layer contains more *smooth muscle fibres, collagen and elastic fibres.*

The *adventitia* contains connective tissue, collagen and some elastic fibres.

The outer regions of the medial layer are supplied by small vessels known as the *vasa vasorum*, whereas the inner layers receive nutrients by diffusion from the circulating blood.

Those arteries near to the heart are known as *elastic arteries*, as they contain more elastic tissue, enabling them to cope with the extreme pressure exerted as the ventricles of the heart contract, ejecting the blood into the circulatory system. *Muscular arteries* are present in the lower extremities of the body, especially in the more superficial areas, which are less well supported. They may also be classified as *conductive* and *distributive* arteries. The former are recognized as arteries which travel straight down the body, e.g. the iliac and femoral arteries; they have few branches. The latter stem from these conductive vessels and form many branches, supplying organs and major tissues of the body, e.g. the superior mesenteric artery and the coeliac artery (Fahey 1994).

Arterial haemodynamics

In simple terms flow through a tube is expressed by

$$Flow = \frac{Pressure}{Resistance}$$

There are a number of factors which influence flow in relation to blood vessels, namely the elasticity of the tubes and the pulsatile nature of the flow.

Blood leaves the heart and passes down the aorta, which is approximately 2 cm

Arterial walls—3 layers:

• intima
• media
• adventitia.

Arteries convey nutrients and oxygen to the peripheral vascular bed.

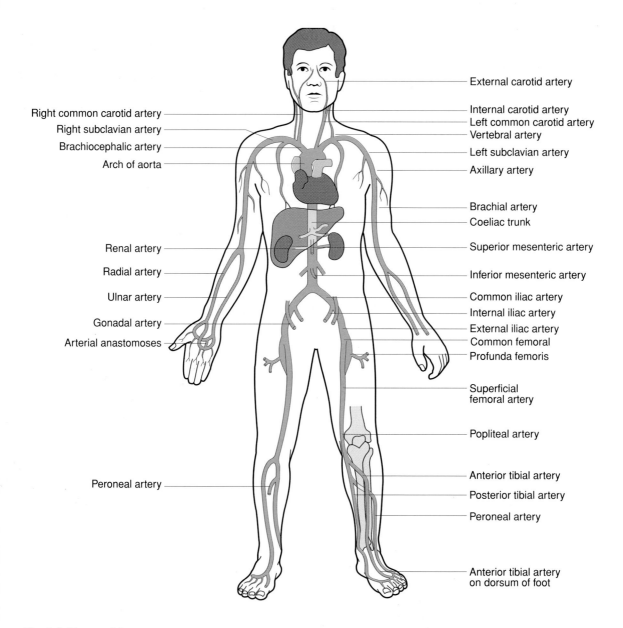

External carotid artery

Internal carotid artery
Left common carotid artery
Vertebral artery

Left subclavian artery

Axillary artery

Brachial artery
Coeliac trunk

Superior mesenteric artery

Inferior mesenteric artery

Common iliac artery
Internal iliac artery
External iliac artery
Common femoral
Profunda femoris

Superficial
femoral artery

Popliteal artery

Anterior tibial artery
Posterior tibial artery
Peroneal artery

Anterior tibial artery
on dorsum of foot

Right common carotid artery

Right subclavian artery

Brachiocephalic artery

Arch of aorta

Renal artery

Radial artery

Ulnar artery

Gonadal artery

Arterial anastomoses

Peroneal artery

Fig. 1.1 The arterial system.

in width. Along the course of the aorta, distributive arteries branch off to major organs and areas of the body, as illustrated in Figure 1.1. The diameter of the conductive arteries gradually decreases as the extremities are reached. For example, the peroneal artery of the leg is approximately 2 mm in diameter.

Arterioles, which are smaller, branch off from the arteries and offer the most resistance to blood flow. As they become capillaries, the resistance becomes less owing to the increase in the total cross-sectional area of the lumen as the number of branches increases and the muscular layer disappears. *Capillaries* permeate into the tissues and allow for the exchange of gases and nutrients, before joining up with the venules and veins which return the blood to the heart.

Any alteration to blood flow will disrupt the balance between oxygen demand and supply. If decreased perfusion, relative to demand, is maintained over a long period of time, the body will set up compensatory mechanisms to ensure that metabolic demands can be met. These may take the form of *vasodilatation*—which on its own has a limited effect, as the vessels are soon dilated to their maximum— and *cellular anaerobic respiration*. In the latter instance the metabolic products which are produced as a consequence, *lactic and pyruvic acid*, will only be excreted slowly by the kidneys, provoking a change in the body's acid-base balance.

> Compensatory mechanisms against impaired circulation
>
> • vasodilatation
> • collaterals
> • anaerobic respiration.

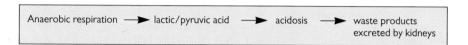

In the long term, the slow development of *collateral vessels* may aid perfusion.

The pulse

Where arteries lie superficially, a pulse can be palpated, e.g. carotid, brachial, radial, femoral, popliteal and pedal—anterior tibial, posterior tibial, peroneal and dorsalis pedis—pulses. There has been disagreement as to whether or not the dorsalis pedis pulse is congenitally absent in 10% of people. However, Brearley et al (1992) demonstrated, using Doppler ultrasound examination, that it was only genuinely absent in 1.9%.

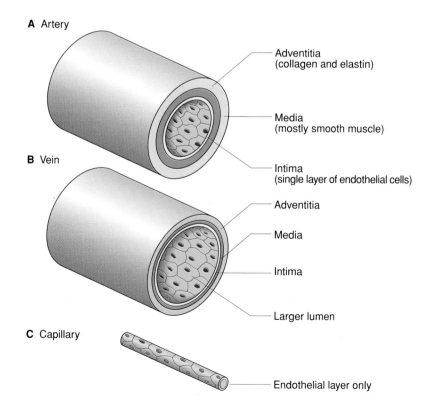

Fig. 1.2 Structure of vessels.

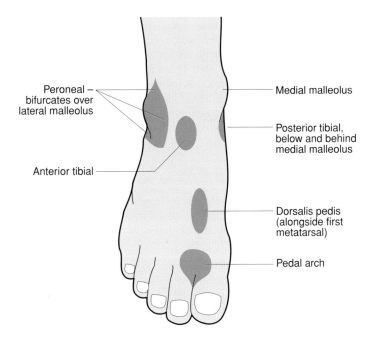

Peroneal – bifurcates over lateral malleolus

Anterior tibial

Medial malleolus

Posterior tibial, below and behind medial malleolus

Dorsalis pedis (alongside first metatarsal)

Pedal arch

Fig. 1.3 Pulses of the foot.

The position of the pedal pulses is illustrated in Figure 1.3.

Where arteries pass over bony prominences in this way, distension can be felt as a rhythmic beat each time the heart ejects 100 ml of blood into the already full aorta. The pulse wave travels at a rate of 7 m per second along the arteries. The *crest* of the pulse wave is recognized as the *systolic pressure* and the *trough* as the *diastolic pressure*. The tension of the pulse is dependent on the blood pressure. Where pulses cannot be palpated at the above sites, they may be audible using a Doppler ultrasonic probe, as described in Chapter 5.

As the blood reaches the inelastic capillaries, it meets with peripheral resistance and the pulse is lost.

> Pulsation disappears when blood reaches inelastic capillaries.

> Blood pressure =
>
> $$\frac{\text{cardiac output}}{\text{peripheral resistance}}$$

Blood pressure

Blood pressure (BP) normally refers to the pressure in the peripheral arteries, unless otherwise stated. It is determined by *cardiac output as ml/min (flow) × peripheral resistance*. An analogy of this is Ohm's law, where voltage = current × resistance.

Peripheral pressure comes under the control of the sympathetic nervous system and cardiac output is controlled by the parasympathetic system (Fig. 1.4).

Cardiac output (ml/min) = stroke volume (ml/beat) × heart rate (beats/min).

Stroke volume depends on:

- Extrinsic factors, which include the effect of noradrenaline and adrenaline on the cardiac muscle. By controlling the entry of calcium into the cells and hence its effect on electrical excitation, these two hormones increase the contractibility of heart muscle fibres.

- Intrinsic factors in accordance with Starling's law of the heart. This law determines that the more the muscles are stretched, the more powerfully they contract—i.e. the more blood that is delivered to the heart, the greater is the volume expelled. It needs to be noted that this is only true within given limits, and if the heart is overstretched heart failure will ensue.

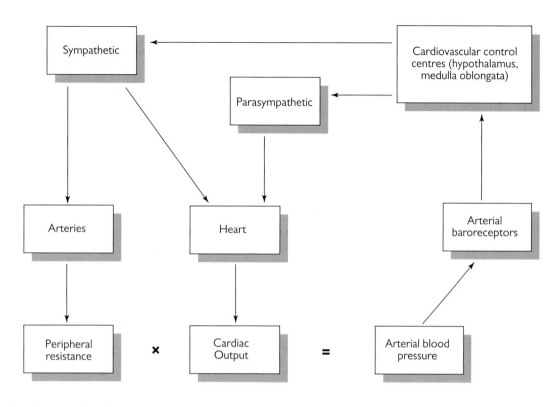

Fig. 1.4 Control of blood pressure.

Factors which influence blood pressure

Baroreceptors are a collection of numerous nerve endings, found in the arch of the aorta and in the carotid sinus at the bifurcation of the common carotid artery. The frequency of nerve impulses varies in order to accommodate changes of pressure in the vessels as they distend at each heart beat. Hence they are sensitive to mean blood pressure and the rate of changes of pressure between each heart beat.

Cardiac output and peripheral resistance are reflexly adjusted in response to the pressure monitored by the baroreceptors. This information triggers adjustments in vasomotor activity originating from the vasomotor centre in the medulla oblongata and transmitted through the sympathetic and parasympathetic nerves. As the mean pressure increases, so does the activity of the receptors, bringing about a shift in the balance between sympathetic and parasympathetic activity, in favour of the parasympathetic system. This results in a reduction in the sympathetic tone of the smooth muscle in the arteries. Heart rate is slowed down in response to the parasympathetic action, which induces a decrease in heart rate and stroke volume. Hence the blood pressure is reduced. If the BP is low, there is an increase in sympathetic action and a decrease in parasympathetic action, resulting in an increase in cardiac rate and stroke volume. In good health, therefore, a stable BP is maintained.

In the normal body the pressure in the arteries of the foot, when supine, should be the same as that in the brachial artery.

In hypovolaemia, the baroreceptors stimulate the sympathetic nervous system to cause vasoconstriction, so counteracting the decrease in blood pressure brought about by, for example, haemorrhage. This sympathetic response accounts for the appearance of the shocked patient who is pale and sweaty, with a tachycardia and reduced urine output.

Factors that influence blood pressure

- baroreceptors
- pharmacological agents: noradrenaline, etc.
- angiotensin
- hyperkalaemia
- prostaglandins
- pain, stress and emotion
- drugs.

Regulation of blood flow

The factors which influence arterial flow are summarized in Table 1.1. Influences which maintain the balance between vasoconstriction and vasodilatation are induced by neural, hormonal and local factors which alter the degree of vasoconstriction and vasodilatation at any one time.

Table 1.1 Factors which influence arterial flow

Physical elements	Circulatory agents	Neurological control	Metabolic influences
Pressure	Prostaglandins	Autonomic nerves	Tension—tissue gas
Ambient temperature	Adrenergic controls	Baroreceptors	Tension—tissue
Atheroma Quantity of blood	Angiotensin Drugs		lactic acid and potassium

Neural factors

The vascular system comes under the control of the *autonomic system*. The *vasomotor centre* (VMC), housed in the *medulla oblongata* in the brain, receives *sensory* impulses which trigger *motor* activity via the *sympathetic nerves* to the smooth muscular walls of the arteries. Vessels are normally held in a state of mild vasoconstriction, i.e. *sympathetic tone*, until they need to respond to changes in the internal and external environment.

Three types of neurones are involved in the transmission of information from the VMC to the vessel walls.

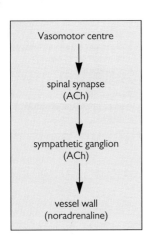

Vasomotor centre
↓
spinal synapse
(ACh)
↓
sympathetic ganglion
(ACh)
↓
vessel wall
(noradrenaline)

1. Messages are transmitted from the VMC in the medulla down the spinal column to the lateral horn cells in the grey matter of the first thoracic to the third lumbar vertebrae.
2. Preganglionic fibres leave the spinal cord via the ventral nerve roots and run to the sympathetic trunk which is parallel to the spinal cord. Acetylcholine (ACh) acts as the neurotransmitter at the ganglionic junction, and therefore these neurones are said to be cholinergic.
3. The postganglionic nerve then passes to the tissue cells. At its synapse with the smooth muscle (the neuromuscular junction), noradrenaline is the neurotransmitter and the neurone is therefore said to be adrenergic. This is illustrated in Figure 1.5. The sympathetic system alone is responsible for neuromotor activity in most vessels. However, the vessels supplying salivary glands and external genitalia also come under the control of the *parasympathetic system* (Green 1992).

Nerve impulses through the sympathetic system are classified by two groups of receptors, alpha and beta. *Alpha receptors* are excitatory, resulting in vasoconstriction, and *beta receptors* are inhibitory, resulting in vasodilatation. Alpha receptors are found mainly in the skin and gut whereas beta receptors are found in skeletal muscle and blood vessels.

Hormonal factors

Adrenaline A hormone produced by the adrenal medulla causing constriction in arteries to the skin and gut, but relaxation in arteries to muscle and vital organs,

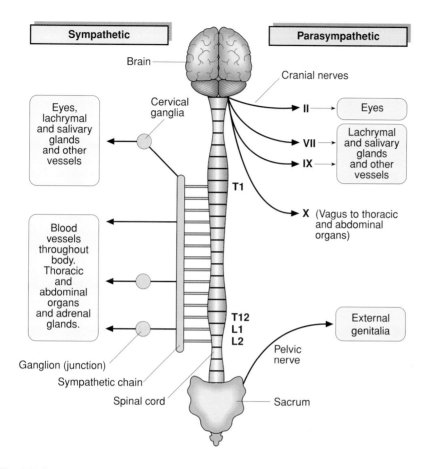

Fig. 1.5 Sympathetic and parasympathetic nerve pathways. Left sympathetic and right parasympathetic nerves, only, shown (both systems are, in fact, symmetrical). Where there is dual innervation stimulation usually produces opposite effects, e.g. sympathetic speeds the heart rate and parasympathetic slows it down.

preparing the body for action. The stroke volume of the heart is increased in response to an increase in adrenaline.

Noradrenaline is produced within the sympathetic nerve endings. It acts as the neurotransmitter at the junction of the postganglionic nerve and the tissue cells as described above. Vasoconstriction and vasodilatation is influenced by the interaction of noradrenaline with the alpha receptors in smooth muscle. Vessels are normally held in a state of tone, but where frequency of the impulses is further increased the extra vasoconstriction brings about a reduction in blood flow. Vasodilatation will enhance blood flow if the frequency of impulses decreases.

Acetylcholine The other neurotransmitter in the sympathetic nervous system, which is also the transmitter in the parasympathetic system.

Kinins are produced from circulating peptides called kininogens by the action of kallikreins. These may be present in the plasma as a product of activation of clotting factor XII, or in tissue. The production of kinins is part of the inflammatory response. Their actions are

• local vasodilatation

- to increase capillary permeability
- to attract leucocytes
- to provoke a pain response.

Angiotensin is a peptide produced when renin is released by the kidney in response to reduced pressure in the renal arteries. This circulates in the blood and brings about *vasoconstriction*. It also produces secretion of aldosterone from the adrenal cortex, which helps retain salt and water, so supporting the blood pressure. If angiotensin is produced in excess it can lead to hypertension (Green 1992).

Prostaglandins In 1930, Kurzrock and Leib discovered a substance in seminal fluid produced in the prostate gland—hence the name 'prostaglandins'. These are tissue hormones which are now known to be synthesized in the endothelial cells and platelets, in the presence of cyclooxygenase, from unsaturated fatty acids which are derived from membrane phospholipids in the diet. They were found to have a relaxing effect on smooth muscle which results in vasodilatation.

There are a number of different prostaglandins which can oppose one another, so affecting:

- Control of vasodilatation or vasoconstriction brought about by, respectively, the relaxation or stimulation of smooth muscle.
- Control of the viscosity of blood. This is an important factor in the management of thrombosis. It is known that acetylsalicylic acid will inhibit the production of cyclooxygenase in platelets, so reducing the aggregation of platelets and consequently their stickiness. Prostaglandin PGI_2 has the same effect, but another prostaglandin, thromboxane A_2 (TXA_2), has the opposite effect, increasing viscosity and also producing vasoconstriction. In a dose of 75–150 mg per day, aspirin reduces viscosity, and this effect may be explained by the fact that PGI_2 is less sensitive to inhibition by aspirin than TXA_2. Prostaglandin PGI_2 may therefore be used as an adjunct therapy following bypass surgery to improve blood flow immediately postoperatively (Gruss 1985).

Local factors

Ambient temperatures At low temperatures, the sympathetic stimuli in the skin result in vasoconstriction of the peripheral vessels in a bid to conserve heat. High temperatures result in vasodilatation as the blood is sent to the skin, enabling heat to be lost from the body.

Gravity In the healthy body gravity has little effect on blood pressure. However, in a diseased limb, the disruption of muscular tone allows gravity to exert an effect on the flow of blood. Patients with arterial disease are often seen with a leg hanging down over the side of the bed at night to assist circulation to the peripheral tissues.

Pain Sensory messages are received by the cerebral cortex (higher centre of the brain), which in turn relays messages to the medulla oblongata, bringing into force vasomotor activity. In moderate pain vasoconstriction will result in a rise in BP. In severe pain vasodilatation results in a drop in BP. This is discussed further in Chapter 4.

Stress and emotion The higher centres of the body transmit messages to the vasomotor centre in the medulla oblongata which evoke the necessary vasoactivity in response to particular situations; for example, vasoconstriction can arise at times of exam stress or a happy family occasion. As the peripheral resistance rises so does the BP. However, should there be a reduction in vasomotor tone or pressure, as seen in overbreathing when the CO_2 becomes insufficient, the BP will fall.

Drugs The effect of drugs, e.g. beta-blockers, will be described in Chapter 13.

Quantity In the case of haemorrhage every attempt is made by the body to maintain pressure by vasoconstriction.

THE MICROVASCULAR SYSTEM

Capillary walls comprise a single-thickness layer of endothelial cells, surrounded by a basement membrane. They form the network between the arterial and venous systems recognized as the *capillary bed*. Capillaries divide profusely, so that all tissue cells are in intimate contact with one. This allows diffusion of molecules of small water-soluble substances such as nutrients, gases and waste products between the tissues of the body and the circulatory system. As the basement membrane is semipermeable, it will not allow the passage of large molecules such as plasma proteins.

The permeability of the capillaries is fairly constant in most tissues, though in some sites there is considerable variation. In the circulation to the brain the capillary pores are small, thus reducing, for example, diffusion of penicillin unless there is meningeal inflammation. This block is known as the *blood–brain barrier*. Treatment for meningitis therefore requires high concentrations of penicillin which will be at their most effective during the inflammatory phase when the pores are expanded; alternatively one can use cephalosporins, which do cross the blood–brain barrier.

In contrast, the capillaries within the liver and bone marrow, the *sinusoids*, have large pores and are almost completely permeable to all molecules, including blood cells and proteins.

Factors affecting permeability of capillary walls

Permeability of capillary walls is dependent on:

- the presence and size of pores between the endothelial cells
- the degree of endocytotic and exocytotic metabolic activity (Rutishauser 1994).

Forces affecting flow of fluid and solutes in and out of capillaries

There are three major forces controlling this:

- *hydrostatic pressure (BP)*
- *osmotic pressure*
- *diffusion gradients.*

Hydrostatic pressure is the pressure exerted by the force of the flow, i.e. the blood pressure (this is much higher at the arterial end of the capillary network).

Osmosis occurs when large molecules cannot pass through a semipermeable membrane and water is attracted across the membrane to the side where there is a higher concentration of large molecules (Fig. 1.6). In the case of blood, there is an osmotic pressure into capillaries because the large plasma protein molecules cannot escape through the membrane. When applied to plasma proteins, this is known as the *oncotic* or *colloid osmotic pressure*. This pressure is much the same at the arterial and venous ends of the capillaries.

The two *forces* act simultaneously, so the effect is a *homoeostatic balance* between the extracellular fluid and the plasma. If the balance is disturbed, for example by high venous pressure, water stays in the extracellular fluid (oedema).

Diffusion occurs when there is movement of a substance from a more concentrated solution to a weaker one (Fig. 1.7). Small molecules such as urea, oxygen, carbon dioxide, glucose, amino acids and electrolytes can diffuse freely across cap-

Pharmacological control of vessel tone

vasoconstrictor substances
adrenaline
noradrenaline
serotonin
dopamine

vasodilator substances
histamine.

Pressures on fluids in capillaries

- Hydrostatic pressure
  diffusion pressure
  for nutrients

- moves fluid out of vessel

- osmotic pressure

- diffusion pressure
  for waste products

- moves fluid into vessels.

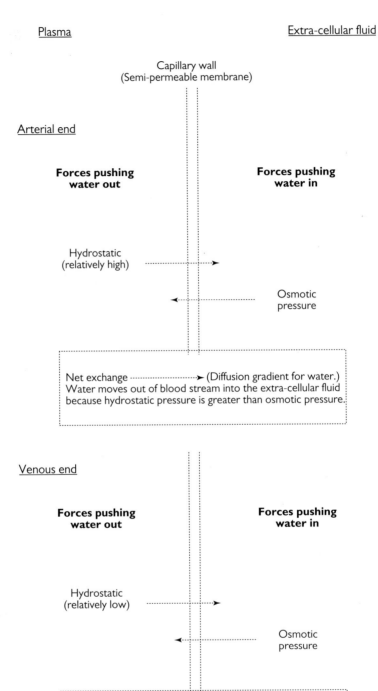

Fig. 1.6 Water exchanges through the capillary wall.

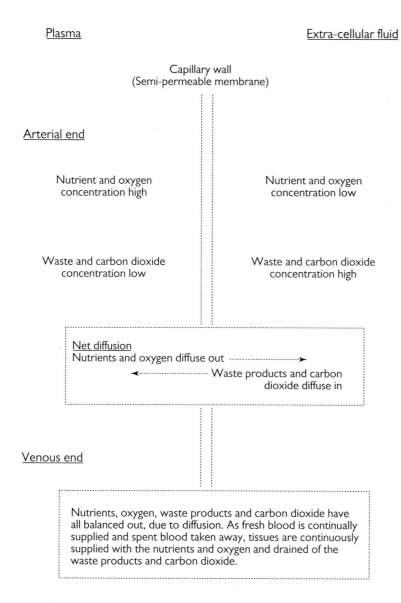

Fig. 1.7 Solute exchanges through the capillary wall.

illary walls. The speed of diffusion depends on the *diffusion gradient*, which is determined by the relative interstitial and endovascular concentrations of the particular substance and by the thickness of the vessel wall.

Other factors affecting blood flow through capillaries

• *The arterioles contain shunts* which can open up in order to bypass the capillaries, for example in a bid to conserve heat (Fig. 1.8).

• Arterioles also contain *precapillary sphincters* (see Fig. 1.8). When muscles are in a resting position, arterioles contract (vasoconstrict) and these sphincters are closed. Blood bypasses the capillary beds of these tissues through the shunts.

Fig. 1.8 Capillary flow.

(A) Active tissue: pre-capillary sphincters open; shunt closed; flow through capillaries high.

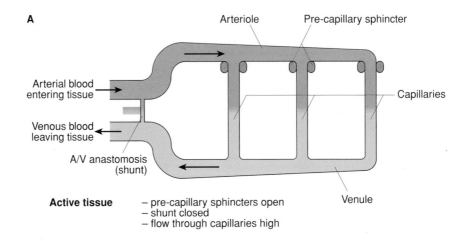

A

Arteriole   Pre-capillary sphincter

Arterial blood entering tissue

Venous blood leaving tissue

A/V anastomosis (shunt)

Capillaries

Venule

Active tissue — pre-capillary sphincters open
— shunt closed
— flow through capillaries high

Fig. 1.8 (B) Inactive tissue: some pre-capillary sphincters closed; shunt closed; flow through capillaries reduced.

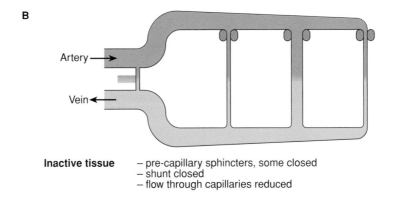

B

Artery

Vein

Inactive tissue — pre-capillary sphincters, some closed
— shunt closed
— flow through capillaries reduced

Fig. 1.8 (C) Inactive tissue conserving circulation (e.g. in low BP states): pre-capillary sphincters closed; shunt open; blood short-circuits capillaries.

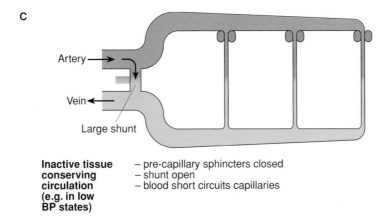

C

Artery

Vein

Large shunt

Inactive tissue conserving circulation (e.g. in low BP states) — pre-capillary sphincters closed
— shunt open
— blood short circuits capillaries

• *A localized increase in metabolites,* e.g. carbon dioxide, in tissue cells stimulates the need for increased blood flow in order to remove these metabolites and replace them with oxygen and nutrients.

It follows that, in certain disease states, blood flow and fluid balances are affected both inside and outside the capillaries.

Haemorrhage In this case the capillaries are constricted and shunts open up (Fig. 1.8). The hydrostatic pressure in the capillaries is therefore reduced, so more interstitial fluid is drawn into the vascular system. Circulating volume is therefore increased and blood pressure is maintained.

Low albumin states, e.g. in poor protein intake or renal failure. Where the concentration of plasma proteins is reduced, the osmotic pressure is also lowered, so fluid tends to stay outside the capillaries in the interstitium. This produces oedema.

THE VENOUS SYSTEM

The venous system (see Fig. 1.9) commences in the capillary beds as capillaries coalesce to form venules. These then unite to form larger single veins. Eventually these become the superior and inferior venae cavae, which return blood to the heart.

The anatomy of veins is not dissimilar to that of arteries, except that they are flat vessels when empty. The medial layer contains fewer smooth muscle fibres, particularly in the deep veins, so making the walls thinner, as illustrated in Figure 1.2. The adventitia is also thicker in the more superficial veins where more support is needed. The intimal layer of the veins is a *multiple layer of endothelium* which is *metabolically active*, producing *plasmin, prostacyclin* and *factor 13*. These enzymes help to prevent the blood from clotting intravascularly. When the veins are damaged the cells of the intima produce serotonin, which brings about vasoconstriction. (Wound repair is discussed later in this chapter.) Larger veins contain a subendothelial layer of supportive tissue to give them extra strength (Wolfe 1992).

The intimal layers contain pouch-like folds—*bicuspid valves*—which open towards the heart, so preventing backflow of blood, especially when the body is in an upright position. The most important valves are at the junctions between the deep, perforating and superficial vessels and prevent backflow of blood from the deep system to the superficial system.

> Endothelial walls of veins produce:
> - plasmin
> - prostacyclin
> - factor VIII.

Veins of the legs

The *venous system* has a *superficial branch* outside the deep fascia—the long and short saphenous veins, which take their name from the Greek *saphenous*, meaning 'to be seen'.

The *deep branch*, which runs parallel to the arteries, is contained within the fascia. Branches of deep veins within the gastrocnemius and soleus muscles can be very large, becoming sinusoidal and so containing large volumes of blood (gastrocnemius and soleus sinuses).

Perforator veins traverse the fascia to connect the two branches (see Fig. 2.7).

Abdominal venous return

In the abdomen, venous blood flows from the superficial veins into the inferior vena cava, which lies behind the peritoneal cavity. Variation in intrathoracic and intra-abdominal pressure influences return. During inhalation blood is drawn from the venous system to the right atrium by the negative pressure in the atrium. During exhalation the reverse occurs and raised pressure in the atrium reduces venous return. Straining on defecation involves trying to exhale against a closed glottis, and hence intrathoracic pressure is increased. This has the effect of reducing venous flow to the heart, and if persistent may contribute to venous hypertension. Backflow into most veins during swings in pressure is prevented by the valves, but there are no valves in the venae cavae.

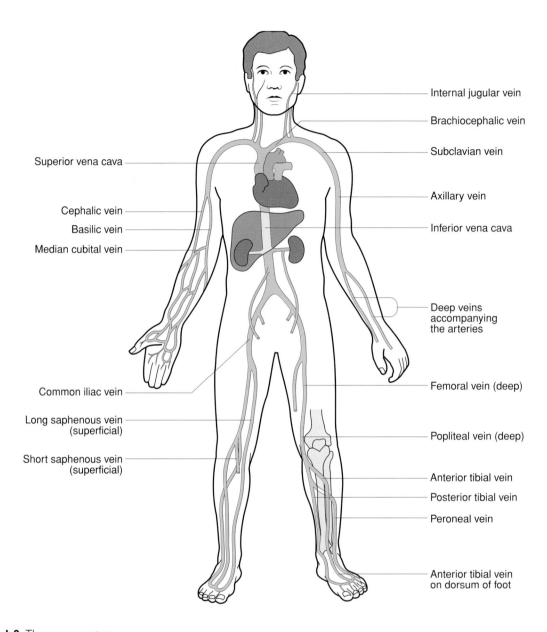

Fig. 1.9 The venous system.

Venous return from the head and neck

Gravity is a major force in helping the return of the blood from vessels above the heart into the superior vena cava, though it opposes the return of blood from dependent parts.

The peripheral veins are richly supplied with sympathetic nerves, which help to maintain a constant body temperature. The *tone* of the veins is also influenced by catecholamines such as adrenaline, noradrenaline and dopamine, all of which mimic the action of sympathetic nerves, as they do in the arteries. The presence of the enzyme *histamine* causes vasodilatation, but that of *serotonin*, an amine present in platelets, causes vasoconstriction. Other drugs—e.g. barbiturates and anaesthetics—induce vasodilatation. Heparin, which is produced by the liver and circulates in the blood, prevents clotting as the pressure behind the venous blood flow is reduced (Fahey 1992).

Venous haemodynamics

Veins are very *compliant*, so allowing them to act as a *reservoir* should blood volume increase quickly, for example during the giving of crystalloids or blood transfusions. As the walls of the vessels distend easily, there is little change in the venous pressure, thus ensuring that central venous pressure is maintained at a constant level under normal circumstances.

Central venous pressure (CVP) is a measure of the pressure in the atria of the heart, which reflects the fluid load in the body.

> The central venous pressure is equal to the pressure in the right atrium.

Regulation of venous blood flow

Factors contributing to the mechanism of blood flow will depend on the position of the vessels in the body.

Venous flow in the legs

During movement the foot and calf muscles exert pressure on the deep veins, so forcing blood to move up towards the heart. This is known as the *foot/calf muscle pump*. In healthy veins, reverse flow is prevented as the intraluminal valves close behind the propelled blood which is returning towards the heart. As the muscles relax and pressure in the deep vessels falls, blood is drawn in through the perforating veins from the superficial system.

> Venous flow in the legs
>
> Downward pressure . . .   due to gravity
> Upward pressure   . . .   due to calf muscle pump.

Normal *venous pressure at the ankle* is around *10–15 mmHg* in the supine position, rising to about *90 mmHg* on standing, equivalent to the height of a column of blood up to the heart. The *ambulatory pressure* in the calf muscles can reach pressures as high as *250 mmHg* on strenuous exercise. During sustained exercise the intraluminal venous pressure drops considerably to about *25–30 mmHg* once the sinusoids have been emptied. It takes approximately 40 seconds to return to normal resting pressure when movement stops (Haeger 1977).

LYMPH VESSELS

These are not dissimilar to veins, except that they contain more valves. Lymph vessels join together to form larger lymph vessels known as *lymphatics*.

Ninety per cent of fluid normally remains in the capillaries, but that which escapes may enter the lymphatic system, through blind-ended vessels which intermingle with the capillaries.

Movement of fluid in the lymph vessels is due to external compression from surrounding muscles.

> The lymphatic circulation depends on muscle compression.

The walls of the vessels contain pores which allow bacteria and debris to enter. Lymph passes through lymph nodes sited in the neck, the axillae, the abdomen and groins. Here, debris and bacteria are phagocytozed. While the lymph from the right arm, right head and neck and right chest drains into the right brachiocephalic vein, the lymph from all of the remainder of the body passes to the cisterna chyli, a

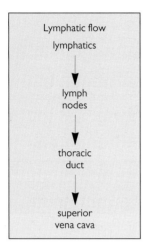

Lymphatic flow

lymphatics

↓

lymph
nodes

↓

thoracic
duct

↓

superior
vena cava

small lymphatic reservoir posterior to the stomach, then rises up the the thoracic duct to drain into the left subclavian vein.

THE COMPOSITION OF BLOOD

The composition of the blood itself has a considerable bearing on the patency of vessels, clotting mechanisms and the healing of wounds. This composition is summarized in Figure 1.10.

Plasma is a slightly alkaline substance (pH 7.4) in which the blood corpuscles float. Its composition is identified in Table 1.2.

Blood gases and pH

The total pressure of the gases in blood may be divided into the partial pressures of single gases. $PaCO_2$ and PaO_2 refer to the partial pressures in the arteries of carbon dioxide and oxygen respectively. The normal partial pressure for *$PaCO_2$ is 3.5–5 kPa* and *for PaO_2 is 11–15 kPa*. The PaO_2 can be reduced to around 10 kPa Hg before the haemoglobin saturation becomes impaired. The normal haemoglobin saturation should be 95–98% (Green 1992).

Carotid and aortic bodies are specialized cells, present in the carotid arteries near the point of their bifurcation and near the aortic arch. They also are supplied by nerve endings from the glossopharyngeal nerve and are sensitive to levels of CO_2 and O_2, initiating reflex adjustments of respiration through the respiratory centre in the medulla oblongata.

An adequate amount of CO_2 is required to allow the vasomotor centre to function properly. CO_2 is a vasodilator to the blood vessels of the brain. If there is a lack of CO_2, for example in hyperventilation, the pH will rise, as CO_2 is an acid. Once it has risen above its normal level of 7.4, the nerves to muscles become more excited, causing vasoconstriction of the blood vessels, a reduction in the blood flow and impairment of vision and dizziness. Variations in pCO_2 and pO_2 act directly on the blood vessels in the brain (*autoregulation*) and do not affect the sympathetic nervous system directly.

Oxygen levels have very little direct effect on the vascular system, except that, where there is a lack of oxygen, constriction of the pulmonary vein may arise; flow through the pulmonary capillaries is consequently slowed in order to maintain oxygen saturation and thereby an adequate supply of oxygen to the tissues of the heart.

CLOTTING

When capillaries are damaged and blood escapes, serotonin is released by the damaged endothelial cells of the vessel walls. This causes vasoconstriction and the clotting mechanism is activated, as illustrated in Figure 1.11. A mesh is formed from fibrin, which is converted from fibrinogen in the presence of:

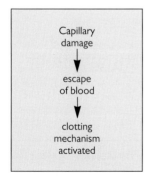

Capillary
damage

↓

escape
of blood

↓

clotting
mechanism
activated

1. calcium salts in the blood
2. prothrombin in the blood
3. thrombokinase found in platelets and damaged tissue.

A clot is formed when platelets become trapped in this fibrin mesh. As the fibres contract, the serum is extruded, so allowing it to dry out. Growth factors known as cytokines are released from the platelets.

Measurement of blood coagulability, e.g. in patients receiving anticoagulants, is discussed more fully later. In brief, it is expressed by laboratories as the *International Normative Ratio (INR)*:

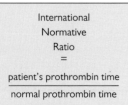

$$\text{International Normative Ratio} = \frac{\text{patient's prothrombin time}}{\text{normal prothrombin time}}$$

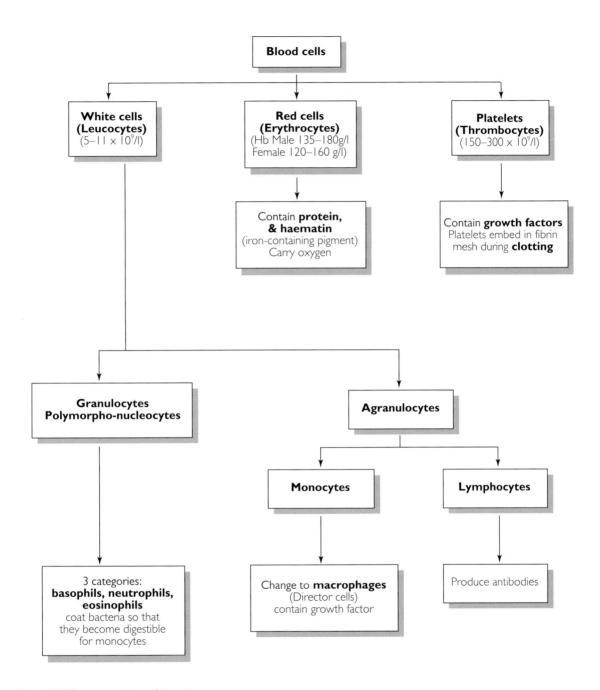

Fig. 1.10 The composition of blood.

Table 1.2 Composition of plasma (normal values will vary slightly from lab to lab)

Proteins	63.00–82 g/l
Serum albumin	39.00–50 g/l
Serum globulin (includes macroglobulin, cryoglobulins, etc.)	24.00–32 g/l
Fibrinogen	1.50–4 g/l
Liver enzymes	
Bilirubin	up to 3.22 μmol/l
Alkaline phosphatase	38.00–126 iu/l
Alanine transaminase	21.00–72 iu/l
Gamma GT	8.00–78 iu/l
Amylase	40–160 units/l
Urea	2.5–6.5 mmol/l
Creatinine	71–133 μmol/l
Salts	
Sodium	136–148 mmol/l
Potassium	3.8–5.0 mmol/l
Calcium	2.0–2.6 mmol/l
Phosphates	38–126 iu/l
Glucose	3–5 mmol/l
Water	90%

Other substances include vitamins, enzymes (including the clotting factors), some antibodies.

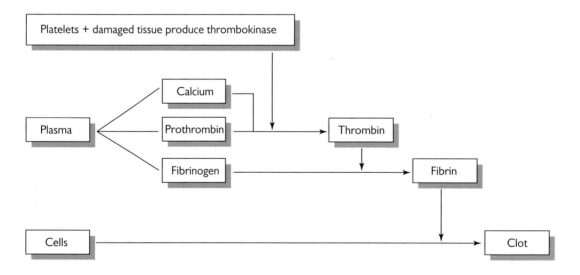

Fig. 1.11 Blood clotting.

SKIN

The skin comprises two layers, the dermis and the overlying epidermis (Fig. 1.12).

The innermost layer of the epidermis is identified as the basal cell layer, which produces keratinocytes that migrate progressively to the outer surface. These produce fibrils of protein known as keratin. During the two weeks that it takes cells to

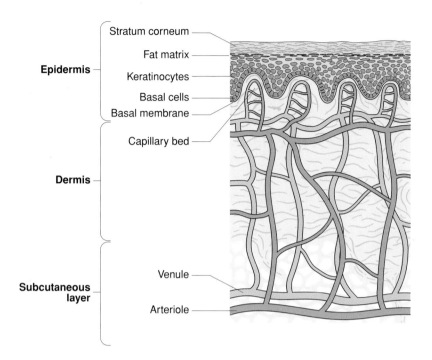

Fig. 1.12 The anatomy of the skin.

migrate from the basal layer to the surface, their content and function changes: they lose their internal structures and become filled with keratin and the protein fillagrin. At the surface the outside layer of the epidermis is known as the stratum corneum. The epidermis contains Langerhans cells, which are defence cells.

The dermal layer contains fibres in between which there are fibroblasts that secrete the proteins collagen and elastin. Collagen gives strength to the tissues and elastin gives skin its flexibility. Also situated in the dermis are sensory receptors, secretory glands, a capillary plexus and many defence cells, including mast cells, which secrete substances involved in the inflammatory process, and histiocytes, which are phagocytic cells.

It is not within the remit of this book to look at all the functions of the skin, but consideration does need to be given to its composition and physiology in order to understand the process of wound healing.

> Skin inactive   . . .   few capillaries
> Skin damaged   . . .   metabolically active   . . .   more capillaries.

Skin is an organ of the body and its functions are illustrated in Figure 1.13.

In healthy skin there is a capillary plexus (network) beneath the epidermis. The basal layer is supplied by small arteries and venules and larger arteries supply the subcutaneous layer.

Should damage occur to the capillary wall, its endothelial layer becomes active in releasing substances which start up the process of wound healing.

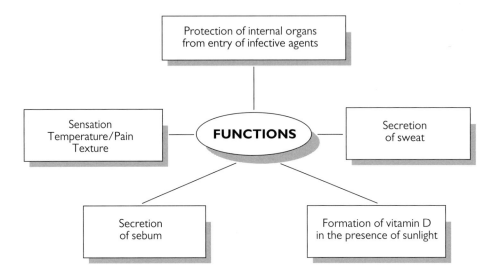

Fig. 1.13 The functions of the skin.

PHYSIOLOGY OF WOUND HEALING

The definition of a wound is *'damage caused to tissue by pressure, shearing, cutting or tearing, burns, frostbite or ischaemia'. Wounds can be found in all soft tissues of the body. They may be created intentionally or accidentally, e.g. by controlled surgical incisions, pressure sores, leg ulcers* (Morison 1992).

Major influences which may adversely affect the healing of wounds are:

- characteristics of the wound
  - the position of the wound
  - haematoma leading to infection.
- characteristics of the patient
  - nutritional state, e.g. low albumin, vitamins A, C, D, B_{12}, iron, magnesium and zinc
  - presence of any congenital tissue disorder, e.g. Ehlers–Danlos syndrome, tumours
  - uraemia
  - skin temperature
  - endocrine disorders, e.g. diabetes
  - ischaemia/hypoxia
  - general health status of the patient, e.g. age
  - allergies, e.g. lanolin
  - immunocompromised patient, e.g. acquired immune deficiency syndrome, leukaemia
  - liver disease, jaundice.
- external factors
  - incorrect nursing management
  - drugs, including tobacco, immunosuppressants and steroids
  - infection
  - chemotherapy
  - foreign bodies, e.g. sutures, prosthetic grafts, chips of bone or splinters
  - patient-controlled factors, e.g. poor compliance, artefactual wounds.

The above need to be taken into consideration in determining the appropriate management of wounds.

Winter (1978) determined that, in order to heal, wounds need an appropriate local environment which must include moisture, warmth and oxygen. In the process of wound healing angiogenesis provides a proliferation of vessels which convey extra oxygen and nutrients to the skin surface. Wounds close in one of two ways, as shown in Table 1.3.

Whichever type of wound closure is involved, a similar healing process occurs. Each phase in the healing process may overlap with the next (Fig. 1.14).

Healing wounds need

- moisture
- warmth
- oxygen.

How wounds close

- primary intention
- delayed
- secondary intention.

Table 1.3 Wound closure

Type of closure (type of wound)	Applied treatment
Primary intention (surgical incision)	Sutures
Secondary intention (ulcers)	Dressings used in leg ulcers

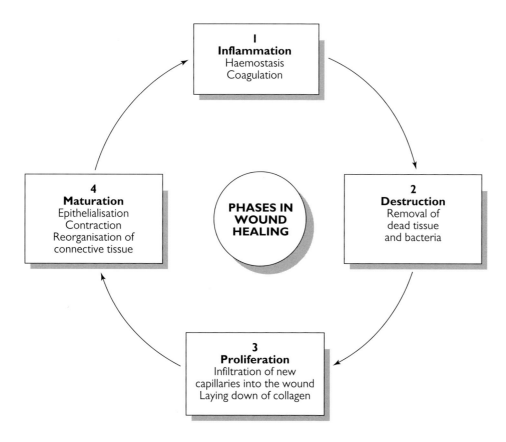

Fig. 1.14 Wound healing.

Stages of wound healing

1. inflammatory
2. destructive
3. proliferative
4. maturation.

Inflammatory phase

As long as it does not get out of hand, inflammation is vital to the process of healing and usually takes 1 to 3 days. However, if it is allowed to continue for too long, hypergranulation of tissues may arise during the proliferation phase. This will also occur if the wound is unable to acquire the oxygen it needs owing to the overuse of occlusive dressings, or the presence of infection.

Maintaining haemostasis

Immediately following trauma to blood vessels a vascular response occurs. Arterioles become dilated and capillary pressure is increased, resulting in accumulation of blood, including large numbers of platelets, at the site of the wound. As endothelial cells have been damaged, serotonin is released. This acts briefly as a vasoconstrictor, thereby controlling the blood loss.

Coagulation

The damaged cells provoke adhesion of platelets to the exposed collagen. This process is known as *platelet aggregation* and results in the initiation of a clot in the wound. Coagulation to produce a mature clot involves the formation of a *fibrin mesh*, which is formed from *fibrinogen*, a serum protein, under the influence of thrombin, as described earlier in this chapter. This mesh traps red and white cells and the mature clot eventually acts as the scaffolding onto which new cells will migrate in the process of tissue repair.

During the inflammatory phase, *mast cells* are released from the endothelial layer. They contain granules of histamine, plus serotonin and leucotonins, which are related to prostaglandins. Histamine promotes vasodilatation, which gives rise to redness, heat and increased permeability of vessels. This increases oxygen and nutrient supply to tissues, but also allows plasma proteins to leak out of the capillary pores, creating an osmotic pressure pulling fluid out of the plasma into the interstitium. Thus localized oedema presents.

During the inflammatory phase pain may arise, owing to the extra pressure in the tissues caused by the oedema. The increased discomfort sensed by the patient may affect movement.

Leucocytes of all types (polymorphonuclear cells, lymphocytes and monocytes) become active in removing damaged tissue, microorganisms and foreign bodies.

Five features may be apparent:

- swelling
- heat
- redness
- immobility
- pain.

Destructive phase

This phase usually lasts 2 to 5 days. The bacteria and tissue debris produce substances which attract *polymorphonuclear cells*, especially *basophils*, which in turn coat the bacteria in a substance that makes them attractive to *monocytes*; these, after ingestion of bacteria and other debris, change to become *macrophages*. Macrophages are often described as the 'director cells' because they are multifunctional. Wound healing can continue when polymorph activity ceases, but should macrophage activity cease wound healing will come to a standstill. In the destructive phase macrophages remove excess fibrin, devitalized tissue and bacteria. In the proliferative phase they stimulate the formation of fibroblasts, which produce the collagen that forms the basis of granulation tissue, and produce a factor that stimulates *angiogenesis*.

Proliferative phase

This process can last 3 to 24 days or longer, depending on the pathological conditions.

Macrophages contain *growth factors*, as do platelets (platelet-derived growth factor—PDGF). Growth factors stimulate tissue revascularization, leading to the formation of new capillaries, or *angiogenesis*. This provides the vascular supply of oxygen and nutrients necessary for the production of granulation tissue. Macrophages also release factors which cause fibroblasts to divide and migrate into the wound. There is now a bed of collagen, which is a structural protein. The wound bed is supplied by newly formed capillaries, which at first are friable and easily damaged.

During this time inflammation subsides and the capillaries produce enzymes which gradually remove the fibrin clot.

Maturation phase

Formation of connective tissue

Fibroblasts continue to migrate from the surrounding tissue and become trapped in what remains of the fibrin mesh, thus producing scar tissue.

The synthesis of collagen by the fibroblasts requires amino acids and proteoglycans for tissue hydration and adhesion. Collagen can only be produced in the presence of vitamin C, iron and oxygen; if these are absent, healing will be impaired. It takes around 120 days for collagen to gain its tensile strength.

Contraction

Some of the fibroblasts change to become *myofibroblasts*, so giving them muscular characteristics, which allow the edges of the wound to be pulled together.

Epithelialization

During this phase, epithelial cells, sebaceous and sweat gland and remnants of hair follicles divide and migrate from the wound edges across the granulation tissue. In a wound closed by secondary intention, epithelial cells migrate from the wound edges and islands of epithelium. When epithelial cells meet, mitosis ceases.

Maturation begins by 24 days but may take *several years to complete* as remodelling takes place. Age and tissue type may influence the rate of maturation. The colour of the scar will fade as the vascularity decreases in the epidermal layer.

REFERENCES

Brearly S, Shearman P, Simms M 1992 Peripheral pulse palpation: an unreliable physical sign. Annals of the Royal College of Surgeons of England 74: 169–171
Fahey V 1994 Vascular nursing. Saunders
Green J 1992 Basic clinical physiology. Medical Oxford Publications
Gruss 1985 Vascular surgery. Baillière Tindall, London
Haeger K 1977 The anatomy of the veins of the leg. From the treatment of venous disorders. MPT Press
Missen J 1975 Principles of intensive care for nurses. Heinemann, London
Morison M 1992 A colour guide to the nursing management of wounds. Mosby, London
Rutishauser S 1994 Physiology and anatomy. Churchill Livingstone, Edinburgh
Wilson K J W, Waugh A 1996 Ross & Wilson: anatomy and physiology, 8th edn. Churchill Livingstone, Edinburgh
Winter G D 1978 Wound healing. Nursing Mirror 146(10): 1–8
Wolfe J 1992 ABC of vascular disease. British Medical Journal, London

Aetiology and pathogenesis of vascular disease

Patients with vascular disorders usually present with the manifestations of end organ damage caused by ischaemia. For example, the kidneys may become ischaemic, resulting in renal failure. Poor vascular supply to the heart may result in angina, or myocardial infarction. Mesenteric artery thrombosis leads to infarction of the bowel. Carotid stenosis may result in visual defects, transient ischaemic attacks or stroke, so causing damage to the brain and nervous system. Poor venous and arterial circulation to the lower limb may result in ulceration of the skin,

---

■ BOX 2.1 Some vascular definitions

Arteritis Inflammation of an artery.
Vasculitis Inflammation of blood vessels.
Angiitis Inflammation of a blood or lymph vessel.
Sclerosis
The hardening of any part from an overgrowth of fibrous and connective tissues, often as a result of chronic inflammation.

Atherosclerosis
The World Health Organization has defined this as a combination of changes in the intima and media, including focal accumulations of lipids, haemorrhage, fibrous tissue and calcium deposits. The development of atherosclerotic lesions is a complex bio-chemical and cellular process. Atherosclerosis in the peripheral arteries, particularly those at the extremities, can severely threaten the survival of tissues.

Thrombosis
The formation of solid from the constituents of flowing blood. The roughened and jagged edges of atherosclerotic plaque encourage the deposition of fibrin in the blood in these diseased areas, providing a mesh on which more platelets can aggregate. The thrombosis may continue to build up until occlusion of the vessel occurs. The enzymes collagenase and elastase, which promote platelet aggregation, are released from the arterial walls as these become irritated by the *turbulent blood flow and stasis*. This acti-vates the clotting mechanism. Eventually the thrombosis may become wide enough to occlude the artery completely and prevent blood flow. *Collateral* vessels may form natu-rally in order to bypass occlusions.

Embolism
Fragments of thrombus, calcified/atheromatous plaque, fat from fractured bones or air may inadvertently be introduced into the vascular system, and circulate as an embolus around the vessels. There is a high risk of an embolus becoming lodged in the branches of the smaller vessels or within major vessels narrowed by atheroma.

Aneurysm
A local dilatation of a vessel, usually an artery.

Vascularization
Development of new blood vessels into tissue.

claudication or limb loss. Deep vein thrombosis may throw off pulmonary emboli, leading to pulmonary infarction. Small vessel disease can have similarly far-reaching consequences.

It is only through taking a careful history and fully investigating the patient's general health and specific symptoms that the underlying vascular disease can be established. Although the vascular disease may be self-evident, care needs to be exercised in elucidating the underlying cause, e.g. infection or diabetes. A holistic assessment of the patient should be made when his or her vascular status is evaluated in order to establish accurate diagnosis and appropriate nursing care.

It is important for the nursing practitioner to have a good understanding of vascular disease in order that symptoms may be observed, recorded and reported to the medical staff to assist them in making a definitive diagnosis.

This chapter aims to provide such an understanding.

ARTERIAL DISEASE

The causes of arterial vascular disease can be divided into two groups, *occlusive disorders* and *aneurysmal disorders*. This chapter aims only to give a brief outline of each situation and does not discuss treatments at this stage. The management of each patient group is discussed under relevant chapters later in the book.

Some of the causes of arterial dysfunction illustrated in Figure 2.1 fall into either *occlusive or aneurysmal* groups. Some may fall into both groups.

> Types of vessel damage
>
> • occlusive
> • aneurysmal.

Occlusive disorders

Virchow identified three factors which increase the risk of intravascular coagulation, and therefore predispose vessels to occlusion (Box 2.2).

Atherosclerosis

The onset of atherosclerosis often dates back to childhood and the early teens. Its progress is divided into three stages:

1. *Fatty streak formation*. These present as yellow thin lines or dots on the intima of arteries and are slightly elevated. At this stage the process is reversible.
2. *Atheroma* can be described as the development of the fatty plaques which appear on the intima, from which atherosclerosis develops. It seldom affects vessels which are less than 2 mm in diameter. There is a loss of elasticity of vessels. The laying down of atheromatous plaques is a variable part of the process of ageing which can be aggravated by smoking and high cholesterol levels. Plaques of atheroma are most likely to form at bifurcations of vessels where there is the greatest turbulence of blood. The narrowing of the vessels will increase pressure locally. If the vessel becomes completely occluded, necrosis of tissues below the narrowing will occur.

■ **BOX 2.2 Virchow's Triad**

1. Change in blood constituents, e.g. platelets
2. Change in vessel walls, e.g. atheroma
3. Change in blood flow, e.g. haemorrhage, heart failure and turbulence.

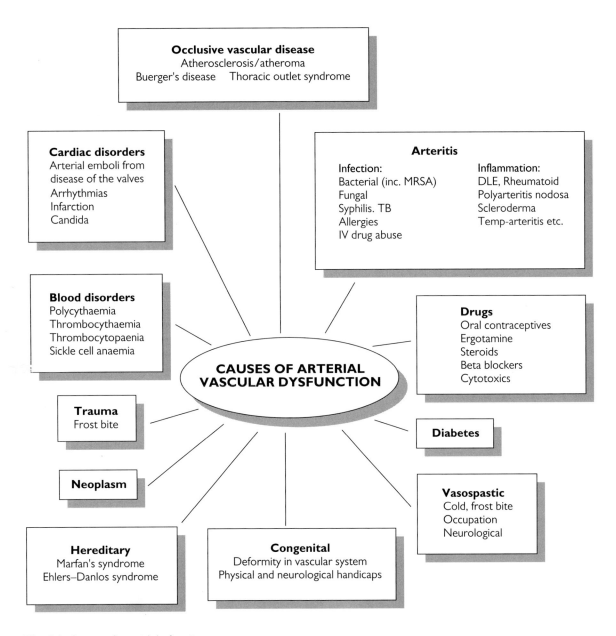

Fig. 2.1 Causes of arterial dysfunction.

3. *Atherosclerosis* (arteriosclerosis). The dictionary defines this as the *changes occurring in walls of arteries that cause hardening and loss of elasticity. Fibrous plaques* form and low-grade inflammation occurs, with a resultant healing response which can leave scar tissue. *Calcification, necrosis and vascularization of* the plaque then develops (Blank 1990).

Figure 2.2 shows a piece of atheromatous plaque which was removed from a carotid artery during a carotid endarterectomy.

Atherosclerosis may cause either occlusive disease or aneurysmal dilatation, owing to the degeneration of the medial lining of the arterial wall. It is the greatest cause of occlusive disease in the Western world, but according to Wolfe (1993) the Japanese have a lower incidence as their diet is not so high in the saturated fat which produces low-density lipoprotein in the blood. Wolfe also states that south-west Scotland and Northern Ireland have a particularly high incidence of athero-sclerosis. However, this anomaly is under investigation by the Scottish Office, which will address issues surrounding peripheral vascular disease and healthy lifestyles.

There are other factors which influence the development of atherosclerosis, namely, cigarette smoking, stress, diabetes, sedentary living, a family history of the disease under the age of 60, hypertension, obesity, hypertriglyceridaemia, hypercholesterolaemia and hyperuricaemia (Fahey 1994).

Hypertension is said to cause atherosclerosis by the deposition of hyaline into the microcirculation from plasma constituents. This is known as hyperplastic arteriosclerosis and raises peripheral resistance (Leitschuh et al 1987). Hypertension by itself does not provoke atherosclerosis; the latter only occurs when hypertension and raised circulating lipoproteins are found together (Chobanian 1983). It has also been shown that people with hypertension have twice the incidence of peripheral vascular disease (PVD), and that with a mild rise in blood pressure there is a raised incidence of claudication (Leitschuh et al 1987).

Hypertension and peripheral vascular disease

- Raised BP + raised lipoproteins = PVD
- Raised BP → hyaline deposition → atheroma
- Raised BP doubles incidence of PVD.

Hyperlipidaemia Where the cholesterol level exceeds the accepted norm of 6.5 mm/l, it is necessary to know the ratio of its two components, high-density and

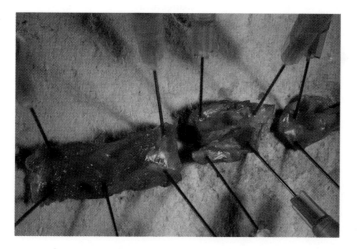

Fig. 2.2 Atheromatous plaque removed from a carotid artery.

low-density lipoproteins (HDL and LDL). Whereas HDLs have a protective effect on the cardiovascular system, LDLs provoke the process of atherosclerosis. An acceptable ratio of HDL to LDL is greater than 0.2.

Conversely, some studies show that very low levels of cholesterol may lead to a higher incidence of depression (Brown et al 1994) and violence (Muldoon et al 1990).

Where there is a combination of the above factors, patients are most at risk of developing serious vascular conditions, e.g. ischaemia of limbs and organs, thrombosis or aneurysm. When vessels are occluded, and the compensatory mechanisms fail, eventually gangrene will ensue.

Buerger's disease, also known as thromboangiitis obliterans

Ninety per cent of cases are men, who are usually under the age of 40. Smoking is the causative factor and the prognosis is usually poor if the patient is unable to stop (Fig. 2.3). However, where the patient stops smoking, the prognosis becomes better than for atherosclerosis.

It is not yet known why cigarette smoking causes such devastating arterial occlusion in some people. However, it is known that nicotine is a vasoconstrictor and some studies suggest that those affected might have an increased sensitivity of the sympathetic system. The vessel walls remain intact, but there is evidence of segmental damage through the layers of the walls. Inflammation can be seen affecting the small and medium-sized arteries and veins. Fibrous tissue and lymphocytes eventually occlude the vessels and enmesh adjacent nerves. The prostaglandin PGI_2 is reduced in patients with Buerger's disease and atherosclerosis, so allowing the viscosity of blood to increase.

The patient first complains of pain in the lower limbs due to claudication, numbness with occlusions in the distal arteries of the lower and upper limbs, thrombophlebitis and ulceration of the toes. If left untreated, the disease may progress to severe states of gangrene, probably as a result of progressive thromboses in the main arteries and collaterals.

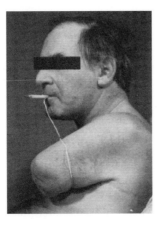

Fig. 2.3 Self-mutilation by smoking: this patient had all four limbs amputated as a result of Buerger's disease. (Reproduced with kind permission from the *British Medical Journal*, from Wolfe (1992).)

Thoracic outlet syndrome

Occlusion of the subclavian artery (1%), subclavian vein (2%) and brachial plexus (97%) can arise when fibrous bands extend from the tip of the transverse process of C7 to the first rib, stretching the lower roots of the brachial plexus (C8–T1). The presence of a congenital cervical rib, abnormal muscle, callus formation following fracture of the clavicle or pressure from enlarged lymph glands and neoplasms may also result in subclavian artery and vein occlusion. Aneurysms can form in the subclavian artery as a result of post-stenotic dilatation. There is a risk of distal embolization from the atherosclerotic changes which form as a result of the continual arterial trauma produced by abnormal structures.

Patients with thoracic outlet syndrome present with pain in the neck, shoulder, forearm and hand; numbness and paraesthesia may also be experienced. Symptoms may be constant or intermittent. In the longer term muscle wasting can be seen in the arms. These symptoms result from an interference with the sympathetic nerve route through the brachial plexus, which lies in close proximity to the abnormal structures described above (Kumar & Clark 1989).

Arteritis

Arteritis usually affects small to medium-sized arteries. The cause may be idiopathic in half the cases, but infections are frequently implicated. Other causes such as autoimmune diseases are discussed below.

The pathogenesis seems to be due to *circulating immune complexes (CICs)* which jam in the arterial walls, provoking an inflammatory response. Polymorphs and damaged endothelial cells invade the lumen and disturbance of blood flow occurs.

> Circulating immune complexes (CICs)
>
> are large antigen–antibody complexes which block arterial wall, producing turbulence in the vessels.

Autoimmune disorders

Giant cell/temporal arteritis and polymyalgia rheumatica These are diseases of the medium to small vessels, associated with high numbers of giant cells (inflammatory cells), monocytes and eosinophils—white blood cells which normally present in higher levels towards the end of the inflammatory phase. The cause of these disorders is not known, but it is thought that they may be due to some underlying malignancy or severe infection.

Histological examination reveals thickening of the intima and necrosis within the medial layer of the artery.

In temporal arteritis, retinal artery thrombosis can lead to total and permanent visual loss, which has been noted in 25% of cases that remain untreated. The patient may present with headaches which are particularly severe in the morning. In the lying position cerebral oedema collects behind the inflammation, causing pressure which can only drain away once the patient is upright. Pain is often experienced along the line of the temporal and occipital arteries, which may also be pulseless. Pain may also be experienced on moving, for example during eating. The skin may become very red over the affected area and, in very severe cases, gangrenous patches may appear on the scalp (Kumar & Clark 1989). The disease is not usually fatal and responds well to a course of steroids.

In polymyalgia, pain is experienced in the muscles in many sites of the body.

Disseminated (systemic) lupus erythematosus This inflammatory skin and organ disease is thought to be an autoimmune reaction to sunlight. It is commonly found in young and middle-aged women, presenting with classical round plaques of hyperkeratosis as a skin rash, possibly over the shins or on the face as a 'butterfly rash'. The *erythrocyte sedimentation rate (ESR)* will be raised. The presence of *cryoglobulins*—proteins in the blood that, when cold, precipitate out of the serum—produces clumps of protein that can occlude vessels. These may be responsible for the secondary complication of Raynaud's phenomenon, resulting in gangrenous digits or elbows and heels if left untreated.

> Important auto-immune disorders
>
> • rheumatoid arthritis
> • disseminated lupus erythematosus
> • polyarteritis nodosa
> • temporal arteritis
> • scleroderma.

Blood disorders

Polycythaemia, thrombocythaemia and leukaemia are blood disorders in which there is an excess of all blood cells, platelets, and white cells respectively. This can result in hyperviscosity of the blood and be a precursor to *thrombosis* and occlusion of vessels.

Disseminated intravascular coagulation is an acquired disorder associated with increased formation of tissue thromboplastin and intravascular coagulation. The process is followed by consumption of platelets, coagulation factors V and VIII, and fibrin, so producing bleeding. This may present following major trauma, blood transfusion, sepsis and ischaemia. Associated clinical signs are acrocyanosis, petechiae and haemorrhage from puncture sites and wounds. Platelet and fibrinogen levels will be reduced, prothrombin time and partial thromboplastin time will be prolonged, degradation products or fibrin splits will be greater than 10 and fragments of red blood cells may be present where normally absent.

Cardiac disorders and arterial emboli

Where *atrial fibrillation* exists, the 'kick' behind the expulsion of blood into the aorta is decreased, giving rise to a potential risk of blood stasis and the formation of thrombus. *Mitral valve disease* also carries the risk of the formation of thrombus as blood stagnates in the left atrium. Following *myocardial infarction*, the formation of secondary ventricular mural thrombi is increased. In cases of *bacterial endocarditis*, the dispersal of microemboli is not uncommon. In these cases, the emboli thrown off may lodge anywhere in the peripheral vessels.

Drugs

These are discussed in more depth in a later chapter. *Ergotamine and beta-blockers* both provoke vasoconstriction with the possibility of occlusion, especially where vessels have already become narrowed by atherosclerosis or calcified plaques in diabetes.

Diabetes

'Vascular disease tends to affect people with diabetes at a younger age and accounts for 75% of deaths in diabetic patients' (Fahey 1994). An increase in *calcification* of the *medial lining* is more common in diabetics. This calcification hardens the walls of the arteries, making them incompressible, so giving inaccurate readings when *Doppler assessment* is used to evaluate the *ankle brachial pressure index (ABPI)*, as described in Chapter 5.

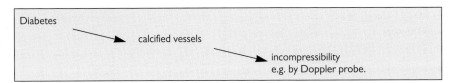

Diabetes → calcified vessels → incompressibility e.g. by Doppler probe.

Diabetic leg ulcers are a complication of a poor vascular supply, neuropathy and a five-fold increase in the risk of infection (Table 2.1). These ulcers often appear on the bony prominences of the feet, with dry, necrotic wound beds, as shown in Figure 2.9 (E).

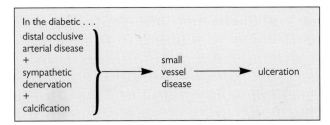

In the diabetic . . .
distal occlusive arterial disease + sympathetic denervation + calcification } → small vessel disease → ulceration

Vascular disease and calcification in diabetics tends to be seen more frequently in the distal popliteal artery and the profunda femoris than in non-diabetics, with an increased risk of small vessel disease.

There is an increased incidence of neuropathy. Diabetic peripheral neuropathy results from ischaemia of the nerves, which in turn is due to poor flow through the supplying vessels, the vasa nervorum. This is related to the degree of glycosylation of the vascular muscle fibres. A loss of sensory nerves puts the patient at risk of trauma created by stepping on sharp objects and pressure from tight shoes. Motor neuropathy leads to unusual pressure exertion on the metatarsophalangeal joints as patients change their gait to maintain balance. This can lead to bone deformities and high pressure on plantar regions of the foot which are unprotected by subcutaneous fatty pads. Callus and ulcers then form. Loss of autonomic nerves leaves the skin of the feet dry, with a high potential for the development of cracks and fissures which may become infected or ulcerate (Table 2.1).

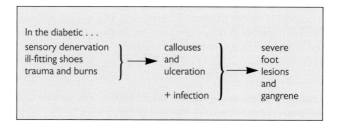

In the diabetic . . .

sensory denervation
ill-fitting shoes → callouses and ulceration → severe foot lesions and gangrene
trauma and burns

+ infection

Table 2.1 Diabetic leg ulcers

Neuropathy	Ischaemia	Infection
Loss of sensory and motor and autonomic neurones	Build-up of atherosclerotic plaque	High blood sugar levels
↓	↓	↓
Paralysis of intrinsic muscles leading to toe deformities, redistribution of pressure	Inflammation of vessels	Fivefold increase in risk of infection
Sensory loss— pressure/trauma		
Loss of autonomic stimulus in vaso-action Loss of sweating		
↓	↓	↓
Ulcer	Ulcer	Ulcer

In diabetic disease arteriovenous shunts may also open because the autosympathectomy reduces the flow of nutrients to the tissues.

Eighty-five per cent of lower limb amputations are performed for vascular disease, a significant number of these being diabetics with occlusive vascular disease (Sooriakumaran 1994). Many diabetics go on to have amputation of a second limb within three to five years of the first, and 60% will die within five years of the first amputation (Fahey 1994).

> - Most amputations for vascular disease are for diabetics.
> - Many diabetic amputees have the other leg removed in 3–4 years.
> - 50% of diabetic amputees die within 5 years.

Neoplasm

Uncommonly, malignant areas of tissue continue to be vascularized. However, the tumour can displace or cause pressure on vessels, resulting in their occlusion.

When the body is cold an autonomic response is for the peripheral vessels to constrict in a bid to conserve heat. This vasoconstriction disrupts both the inflow and the outflow, so preventing the exchange of nutrients and metabolic wastes. In severe cold, the extracellular fluid freezes and crystallizes, so increasing its sodium concentration. Cells become dehydrated as the intracellular fluid moves out in order to maintain homoeostasis. The cell walls consequently rupture and histamine is released, so increasing capillary permeability and resulting in oedema. The red blood cells clump in the capillaries and small blood vessels, causing stasis and occlusion. If the cells cannot be quickly reperfused, cell necrosis will progress to permanent loss of function and gangrene. Tissue trauma may also arise owing to direct thermal damage.

Vasospastic disorders

There are many causes of vasospastic disorders. These may be identified as being associated with trauma, frostbite, emboli, occlusive disease, systemic conditions, e.g. myxoedema, ergotism, cryoglobidonaemia, agglutinism, cold haemagglutination, macroglobulinaemia, collagen disorders such as scleroderma, occupational repetitive strain such as piano playing, typing or working with vibrating machinery.

> Cryoglobulins are proteins which solidify in the cold, blocking small vessels.

Raynaud's phenomenon, described by Maurice Raynaud in 1874, presents as a recognised series of events and 90% of cases seen are in women. When sufferers are exposed to cold or emotional stress the digits suddenly become pale, followed by cyanosis and then erythema. This is because, initially, the tissue is deprived of blood as vessels become constricted. There follows a period of sluggish return of flow and, as this blood is not fully saturated with O_2, the digit is cyanosed. As flow returns to full capacity there is a reactive hyperaemia and digits become erythematous and painful. This colour sequence helps to distinguish Raynaud's phenomenon from acrocyanosis and livedo reticularis.

Acrocyanosis This primarily presents in women between the ages of 15 and 35. There is continuous diffuse cyanosis, usually in the hands but occasionally in the feet. Ulceration does not usually arise, though presenting signs are increased on exposure to cold. Pain, numbness and coldness may inhibit activities which involve use of the hands.

Livedo reticularis Men and women may be affected by this condition at any age. The skin presents with mottled cyanosis or rubor. It is more usually found in the lower extremities of the body, but may appear in the arms. Ulceration is rare, but the symptoms are continual. The patient may experience pain, numbness and a feeling of coldness.

Vibration may be an occupational hazard and Raynaud's phenomenon is often seen in people working with hand-held machines such as sanders and pneumatic drills.

Patients presenting with thoracic outlet syndrome and collagen disorders, who give a history of joint pain (arthralgia), dysphagia or dry mouth (xerostomia), should also be considered to be at risk of Raynaud's phenomenon.

Physical handicaps may affect the sympathetic tone of vessels, resulting in vasospasm.

Sudeck's atrophy Following fracture in any bone, or hip replacement, the sympathetic nervous supply to the lower limbs may become damaged. This may result in vasoconstriction, ischaemia and ulceration of the lower limbs.

Aneurysm formation

Knowledge of aneurysms goes back as far as the second century A.D., when Galen described an aneurysm as 'A localized swelling with pulsation, from which if punctured, bright blood spurted with much violence' (Erichsen 1844). In 1757, William Hunter classified aneurysms as *true or false*, and this classification remains in use today. A true aneurysm occurs when the layers of arterial wall become distended and thin, yet remain intact. The formation of aneurysms is usually due to inflammation that weakens the integrity of vessel walls, rather than pressure exerted on them. Thrombus may be able to collect between the layers of the vessel wall, causing a local dilatation (Fig. 2.4 (A), (B) and (C)). In the case of a false aneurysm, trauma to all three layers of the arterial wall allows seepage of blood extravascularly, and clot formation occurs around which periarterial connective tissue is laid down (Fig. 2.4 (D)). Arterial blood can then flow into the scar sac as it passes along the lumen of the vessel. Thrombus may collect, so increasing the pressure on the arterial wall, leading to a potential risk of rupture (Greenhalgh 1990).

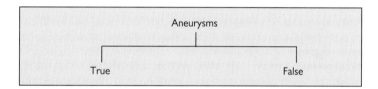

Aneurysms can arise in any artery, but they are most frequently found in the abdominal aorta. They may well go unnoticed unless they are picked up inadvertently during scanning for another reason, or in a screening programme. Occasionally, the patient may present with minor symptoms such as an ache in the back, abdomen or legs.

Men are five times more likely to present with an aneurysm than women, and the incidence is higher in white ethnic groups than in black (Fowkes 1990). In the early stages, aneurysms tend to grow at a rate of around 0.5 cm in width per year. The rate of growth may steadily increase as they become larger. Currently there are studies under way seeking to determine the optimum time for elective surgery. Some schools of thought suggest that aneurysms may safely be left until they reach 5 cm in width while others favour surgery on aneurysms of 3.5–5 cm. Where it is possible to operate on an aneurysm under controlled conditions the mortality is less than 5% (Sooriakumaran 1994).

Causes of aneurysms

Degeneration

This may be found in the medial lining of the arterial walls. It may be congenital or it may arise owing to ageing of the vessel walls.

Aneurysms

Epidemiology

- males > females
- caucasian > Afro-Caribbean

Surgical assessment

- growth 0.5 cm (width) per year
- indication for surgery: width > 5 cm
- ELECTIVE surgery mortality <10%.

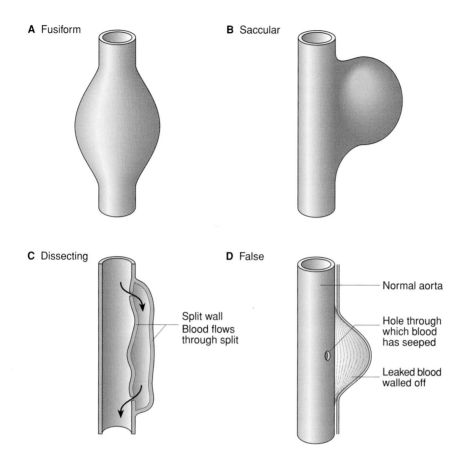

Fig. 2.4 Types of aneurysm.

Infection

Whether the source of infection is localized or systemic, as pathogens become lodged in the normal vessel wall or within artherosclerotic plaques, weakening of the structures will occur which may result in the formation of an aneurysm. It is the thoracic aorta which is most likely to be affected following tuberculosis or syphilis.

Hypertension

From screening programmes in the UK it is known that, in 10% of patients, hypertension may also be a feature in the formation of aneurysms.

Drugs

Some drugs may have the effect of weakening the vessel walls, making them susceptible to aneurysm formation. *Corticosteroids* reduce the integrity of the vessel walls and may result in aneurysmal defects in larger vessels, as well as capillary haemorrhage.

Inflammation

Unknown cause Medial degenerative changes are characterized by dystrophic calcification of the medial lining of arteries, especially in the elderly and those with diabetes. It is mainly the lower limb arteries which are affected.

Collagen disorders resulting in inflammation All these conditions will present with a raised ESR or CRP (C-reactive protein). The laying down of excess collagen narrows the lumen of the vessels.

Temporal arteritis This was discussed above, as it also causes occlusive disease. Occasionally a dissecting aortic aneurysm will form.

Polyarteritis nodosa This tends to affect men twice as frequently as women and presents at around the age of 50. It is a systemic disease in which necrosis of the fibrin in small and medium vessels results in microaneurysm formation. The patient may present with progressive failure of the organs of the body and the prognosis is poor.

Takayasu's syndrome, otherwise known as *Martorell's syndrome* or *pulseless disease,* is most prevalent in Japan. It is of unknown cause, but there are some suggestions that the aetiology is either autoimmune or related to tuberculosis. It mostly affects large vessels, e.g. the aorta at the site of the aortic arch and the abdominal aorta. It is a collagen disease affecting mainly women from the age of 10 to 30 who present with anorexia, night sweats, general malaise, pyrexia and weight loss. Hypertension and eventual cardiac failure may result. Histological examination demonstrates widespread sclerosis and destruction of the elastic fibres in the inflamed medial lining of the arterial wall, plus the presence of giant cells and lymphocytes. Areas of stenosis and saccular aneurysms arise along the length of the aorta and its branches (Robbs 1990).

Unusual forms of vasculitis that can lead to aneurysm are shown in Table 2.2.

Inherited collagen disorders

Marfan syndrome This was described by Marfan, a French paediatrician, in the late nineteenth century, and is characterized by elongation of the skeleton and asymmetry of the face. Degeneration of the medial lining leads to the formation of a dissecting aneurysm, usually in the ascending aorta. The cause is unknown (Leitschuh et al 1987).

Ehlers–Danlos syndrome This is characterized by velvety skin which is hyperextensible, but shrinks normally after stretching. Wound healing may be poor, and leave scars. Bruising occurs very easily, as blood vessels are very fragile, and occasionally an aortic aneurysm develops, which is vulnerable to rupture.

Other factors These include congenital deformities and trauma to vessels. Cytotoxic drugs and steroids make vessel walls thin and therefore prone to aneurysm.

Table 2.2 Unusual forms of vasculitis that can lead to aneurysm

Cogan's syndrome	Kawasaki's disease	Behçet's disease	Drug abuse
Affects large vessels and muscular arteries	Affects small children	Inflammation of iris and ciliary body	Necrosis of artery
May result in deafness, systemic vasculitides, heart failure and haemorrhage, intravascular keratosis	Acute pyrexia Inflammation of coronary arteries, arrhythmias and infarcts	Ulcers (mouth/genitalia, systemic) DVTs Occasional aneurysm	Inadvertent piercing in administration of i.v. drugs

VENOUS DISORDERS

Causes of venous disorders are summarized in Figure 2.5 and discussed below.

Should valves in the lumen of the veins become *traumatized* or be *congenitally absent, backflow* and *stasis* of venous blood increase the pressure on the vessel walls, resulting in *venous hypertension*. This in turn results in tortuous veins and possible ulceration (Fig. 2.6).

During the *menopause* and in *pregnancy, hormones* affect the tone of vessels, causing them to be more relaxed and dilated. In pregnancy the weight of the fetus and increased uterine fluid and blood flow increase intraluminal pressure on the valves in the veins, leading to further distension and weakening.

Occupations which involve much standing put high demands on the valves. With the normal *ageing* process, *degeneration* of valves may lessen their effectiveness. Incompetent veins can be hereditary.

Phlebitis is inflammation of a vein, usually due to infection or trauma. It may be *superficial* or *deep*.

Abnormalities of flow and damage to the endothelium encourage thrombus formation, leading to *thrombophlebitis. Superficial and deep venous thrombosis* occlude vessels. New vessels (*recanalized*) known as *collaterals* form without valves, and *venous insufficiency* arises. The veins become less capable of returning blood to the heart and, as it stagnates in the venous reservoirs, so the risk of *thrombosis* formation and *pulmonary emboli* increases.

Antithrombotic agents

The smooth luminal endothelial layer within the veins and arteries produces antithrombotic factors, *protein C and protein S*. These are enzymes that inactivate clotting factors V and VIII, so reducing the risk of intraluminal clot formation. This is especially important in the veins, where the velocity of blood flow is less than in the arteries and where there is a risk of venous stasis due to incompetent valves.

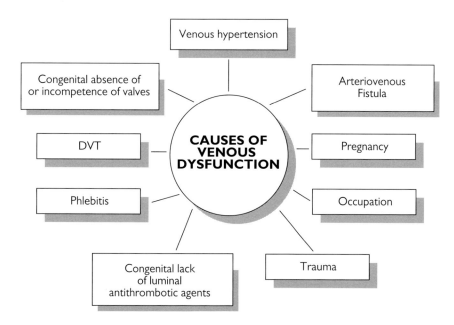

Fig. 2.5 Causes of venous dysfunction.

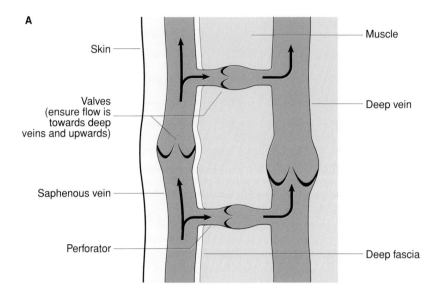

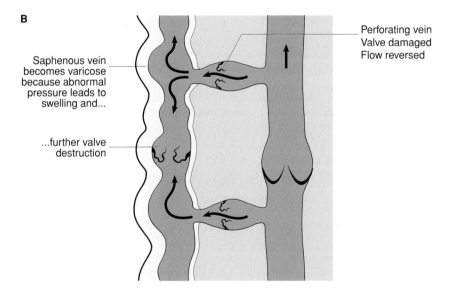

Fig. 2.6 The formation of varicose veins. **(A)** The normal vein: competent valves propel blood upward and inward. **(B)** A varicose vein.

However, should trauma to the vessels occur, interference with this mechanism may arise, and there are also problems in the rare conditions characterized by a congenital lack of these antithrombotic proteins. Platelets aggregate around the damaged area and fibrin entraps circulating red and white blood cells and additional platelets, so producing a clot. Thrombus may collect at the site or become embedded in the angle behind the open valves, so increasing backflow pressure and damage to the valves themselves. *Fibrinolytic activity* may help to reduce the risk of clot formation, unless there have been several episodes of idiopathic deep vein thrombosis, in which case fibrinolysis is reduced.

Pulmonary embolism (venous emboli)

In 90% of cases, the deep veins of the legs and pelvis are found to be the source from which the embolus originated (Rosenow et al 1981). An embolism is an intravascular solid comprised in 99% of cases of thrombus. Circulating air, bone marrow, fat, vegetation from the cardiac valves in endocarditis, septic thrombi and amniotic fluid may also be responsible for an embolic episode. In association with lung cancer, fragments of tumour may embolize.

Emboli travel back through the heart via the peripheral veins and become lodged in the pulmonary artery, causing partial or complete blockage. Hume et al (1970) have suggested that it would take a considerably large embolus to occlude the pulmonary artery and that evidence supports the view that occlusion is exacerbated by intravascular reaction. Serotonin, histamine and catecholamines are released by the endothelial lining of the vessels in response to the platelet degranulation that arises during pulmonary embolism. This results in vasoconstriction of the pulmonary arterioles and bronchoconstriction, placing a strain on the pulmonary vasculature. To restore the previous level of blood flow through the lungs, the right ventricle is required to work harder against an increased resistance, a task for which it is not designed. This may therefore result in pulmonary hypertension or right ventricular failure, with a consequential reduction in cardiac output, leading eventually to collapse (Hume et al 1970).

Chronic pulmonary hypertension

This may result in hypertrophy of the right ventricle following several small episodes of pulmonary embolism.

Varicose veins

The vessel walls become stretched and tortuous, i.e. *varicozed*, as the incompetent valves allow blood to back flow, so dilating them and altering the normal pressures (Fig. 2.6).

Varicose veins fall into two groups, primary and secondary. In the presence of primary varicose veins, the ambulatory pressure drop within the veins is the same as in the normal leg, as described in Chapter 1; however, refilling takes longer. In the presence of secondary varicose veins, the ambulatory pressure drop is less than in the normal vein and is dependent on the venous damage (Hobbs 1993).

As the superficial veins become varicozed, they may cause cosmetic concern. The patient may complain of heavy, aching legs, which become tired and swollen.

Box 2.3 summarizes the features of primary and secondary varicose veins.

Fig. 2.7 Primary varicosis. (Reproduced with kind permission from Medi Stumpf.)

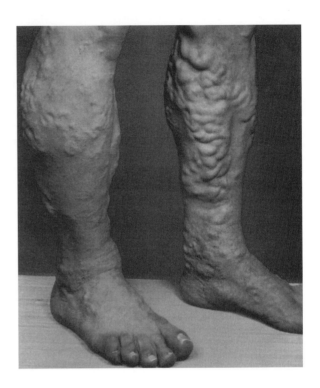

Venous ulcers

Currently there are three theories underpinning venous ulcers as outlined in Figures 2.8 (A, B and C).

Small capillaries may initially be protected against high venous pressure in the legs by the fibrin cuffs, as the process of leg ulceration is seen to be reversible when venous hypertension is reduced. Whilst these theories are accepted, it is suggested that changes in the deep venous system are of primary importance to the secondary changes in the microvascular system (Burnard et al 1982).

Venous ulcers are usually found within the gaiter area, i.e. from mid calf to below the medial malleolus. There may be small ulcers scattered over this region or one large and shallow ulcer with dependent oedema, which makes it feel hard around the edges. Immobility and obesity will aggravate ulceration. Seventy per cent of leg ulcers are found to be of venous origin (Cullum et al 1995).

Primary varicose veins

- usually present with family history
- weakness in medial layer of the vein wall
- Incompetence of valves

Secondary varicose veins

- following DVT
- presence of arteriovenous shunt
- trauma following surgery, shearing, tearing and penetration.

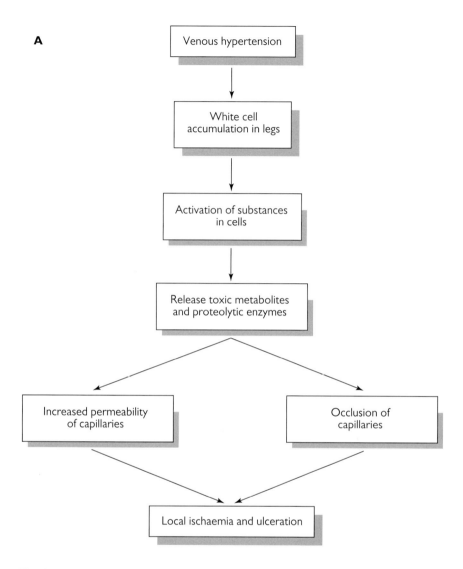

Fig. 2.8 Theories on the genesis of venous ulcers. **(A)** White cell trapping theory. (After Coleridge et al 1988)

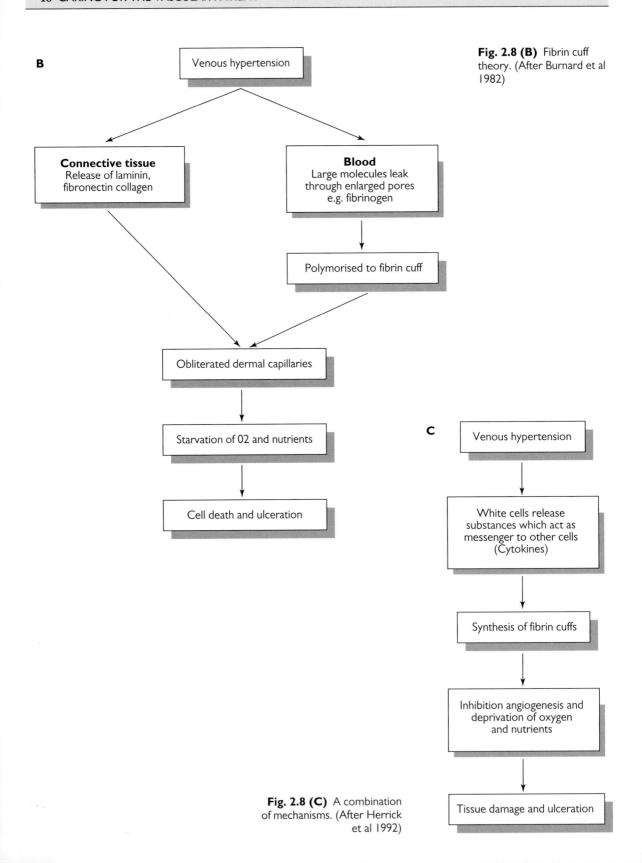

B

Venous hypertension

Connective tissue
Release of laminin,
fibronectin collagen

Blood
Large molecules leak
through enlarged pores
e.g. fibrinogen

Polymorised to fibrin cuff

Obliterated dermal capillaries

Starvation of 02 and nutrients

Cell death and ulceration

Fig. 2.8 (B) Fibrin cuff
theory. (After Burnard et al
1982)

C

Venous hypertension

White cells release
substances which act as
messenger to other cells
(Cytokines)

Synthesis of fibrin cuffs

Inhibition angiogenesis and
deprivation of oxygen
and nutrients

Tissue damage and ulceration

Fig. 2.8 (C) A combination
of mechanisms. (After Herrick
et al 1992)

Causes of venous ulceration

The causes of venous ulceration are summarized in Figure 2.8.

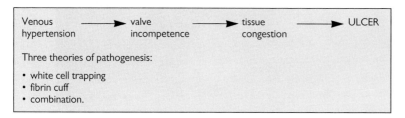

Galen stated that ulcers were for 'the release of foul humours from the body'. Today we aim to heal ulcers of any aetiology as soon as possible. Being able correctly to identify the cause will influence the efficacy of the treatment.

Venous hypertension will result in extra pressure on the walls of the capillaries, which are only the thickness of a single epithelial cell. This pressure creates stretching of the cell walls, and the pores between the cells become enlarged, so allowing abnormal leakage into the skin tissues of oedema and breakdown products from blood.

This may result in the formation of:

Brown staining of the skin, as *haemosiderin,* an iron-carrying pigment present in the haem, is squeezed out of the red blood cells which become trapped in the capillary beds (Fig. 2.9 (A)).

Varicose eczema due to irritation of tissues by the breakdown products of blood. As the capillary beds become congested the dermal layer is starved of oxygen, so preventing cells from maturing. The body strives to bring mature cells to the epidermal layer, and as a result there is an overproduction of cells, which present as eczematous scales (Fig. 2.9 (B)).

Oedema, as the plasma proteins and water are lost from the capillaries to the tissues.

Secondary to venous incompetence and hypertension, *lipodermatosclerosis, venous ulcers* and *eczema* may present as seen in Figure 2.9. In lipodermatosclerosis tissues become thickened, indurated (hardened), eczematous and stained. Ankle oedema, atrophie blanche or ankle flare may also be present.

By comparison, *arterial ulceration* results from tissue deprivation of oxygen and essential nutrients due to arterial occlusion, usually caused by atherosclerosis. Waste products cannot be removed and become toxic to the tissues. These ulcers are normally sited on the foot, especially around pressure points. Arterial ulcers make up around 27% of all ulcers that present.

The leg may be cold and pale, blanching when elevated and only slowly recovering its colour when supine (sunset leg). The skin of the leg may be shiny and hairless owing to a lack of nutrient diffusion to the tissues from the poor blood supply. Some atrophy of the calf muscles may be evident and toenails may have atrophied. Arterial ulcers are often painful, especially at night. They are described as having a 'punched out' appearance and may present with tough adherent slough. Healing is slow because of the underlying ischaemia, unless this can be reversed. Factors contributing to arterial ulcers are summarized in Figure 2.10 on page 53.

Twenty per cent of ulcers are of mixed aetiology, i.e. they have a venous and an arterial component (Fig. 2.9 (D)).

Other causes of leg ulcers are vasculitis-associated inflammatory disorders—e.g. rheumatoid arthritis, DLE, scleroderma or polyarteritis nodosa—malignancy, metabolic disorders, haemolytic disorders, and diabetes as discussed above (Fig. 2.9). These ulcers are further defined in Table 2.3, which highlights the characteristics that enable a differential diagnosis to be made, and illustrated in Figure 2.9.

Causes of venous hypertension

- obesity
- pregnancy
- abdominal pressure
- previous DVT.

Causes of arterial ulcers
Poor perfusion of oxygen

- occlusion
- vasospasm
- small vessel disease
- haemolysis
- Buerger's disease
- Sudeck's atrophy.

Fig. 2.9 Types of leg ulcer.

Fig. 2.9 (A) Varicose veins and venous ulcer.

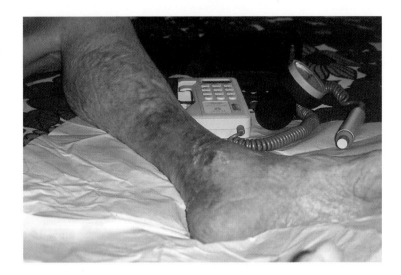

Fig. 2.9 (B) Venous lipodermatosclerosis. Gaiter region of leg.

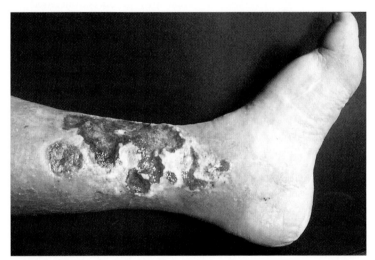

Fig. 2.9 (C) Arterial ulcer: often presents on the foot, with a round, 'punched out' appearance.

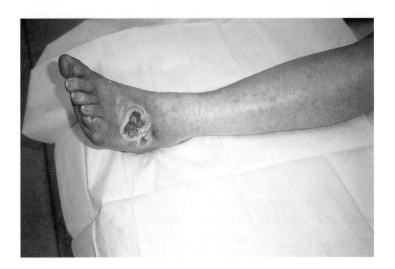

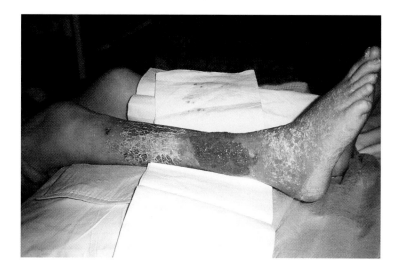

Fig. 2.9 (D) Mixed arterial and venous ulcer: note overgranulation due to presence of infection.

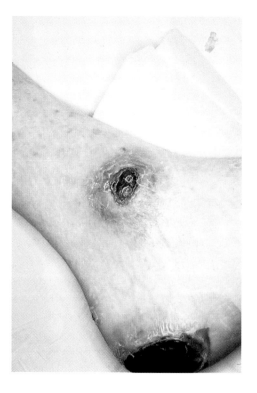

Fig. 2.9 (E) Diabetic ulcer: sympathetic neuropathy; dry necrotic wound bed.

Fig. 2.9 (F) Rheumatoid ulcer associated with inflammation of small vessels.

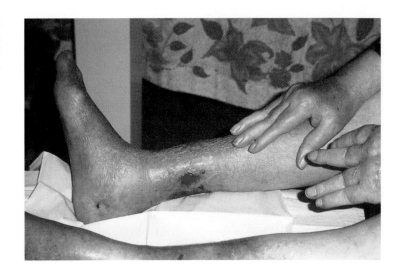

Fig. 2.9 (G) Squamous cell malignant ulcer.

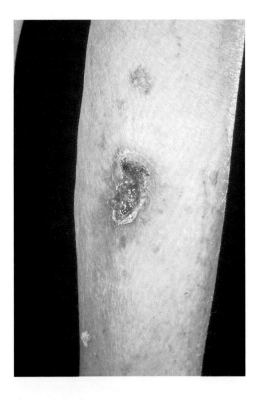

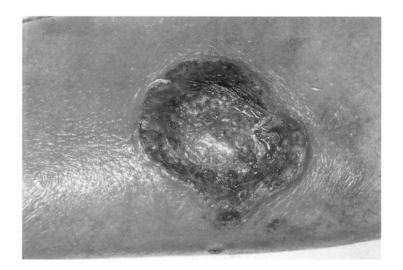

Fig. 2.9 (H) Pyoderma gangrenosum: metabolic ulcer.

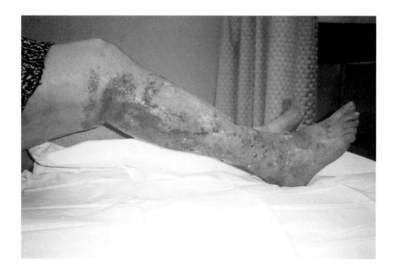

Fig. 2.9 (I) Skin allergy in a patient with an arterial ulcer, following use of a primary dressing.

Table 2.3 Differential diagnosis for leg ulcers

	Venous	Arterial	Diabetic	Rheumatoid	Malignant
Site	Gaiter	Any part of leg, more commonly on foot	Any part of the leg, commonly below the ankle and on the foot	Any part of the leg	Anywhere on the leg
Size	Usually large	Usually small	Often small	Often small	Continues to grow
Edge	Shallow with diffuse edges, irregular	Punched out— deep with cliff edges	Deep with cliff edges	Cliff edges, punched out	Rolled, cauliflower
Exudate	Exudating	Dry	Dry	Dry	Exudating or dry
Oedema	Generalized	Localized	Localized	Localized	Localized
Surrounding skin	Usually brown, presence of lipodermato- sclerosis or varicose eczema	May have dependent rubor, pallor or cyanosis; shiny, hairless	As for arterial; deformities of bone and gait; loss or altered sensation in feet	Bone deformities	None
Varicosity	Sometimes	Only in presence of mixed venous and arterial disease	None, unless mixed with venous disease	None, unless mixed aetiology	None
Pain	Some	Very painful, especially at night	Hyper- or hypo- sensitive, dependent on degree of denervation	Painful	Not usually
Blood profile	Possible reduction in serum albumin			Raised ESR or rheumatoid factors	?Raised ESR
Pulses	Normal	Reduced/absent monophasic signal	Reduced or absent	Reduced	Normal
Doppler ABPI	> 0.8	< 0.8	Reduced or falsely elevated; > 1.4 in presence of calcified vessels	May be reduced to < 0.8 *or* falsely elevated owing to inflammation	0.9–1.2

REFERENCES

Blank I 1990 Nursing Clinics of North America 25: 777–794

Brown S L et al 1994 Low cholesterol concentration and severe depressive symptoms in elderly people. British Medical Journal 301: 1328–1332

Burnard K et al 1982 Pericapillary fibrin in the ulcer-bearing skin of the leg; the cause of lipodermatosclerosis and venous ulceration. British Medical Journal 285: 1071–1072

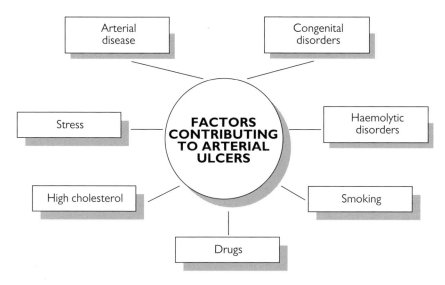

Fig. 2.10 Factors contributing to arterial ulcers.

Chobanian A 1983 The influence of hypertension and other haemodynamic factors on atherosclerosis. Proc Cardiovascular Disease 26: 177

Coleridge et al 1988 Causes of venous ulceration; a new theory. British Medical Journal 296: 1726–1727

Cullum N et al 1995 Leg ulcers: nursing management. Scutari, Middlesex

Eastcott H 1973 Arterial surgery. Pitman Medical

Erichsen J 1844 Observations on aneurysm. London

Fahey V 1994 Vascular nursing. Saunders, London

Fowkes 1990 Prevalence of aortic aneurysm. In: Greenhalgh R, Mannik (eds) The cause and management of aneurysms. Saunders

Greenhalgh R 1990 The cause and management of aneurysms. Saunders

Hallet J et al 1995 Patient care in vascular surgery. Little, Brown, Boston

Herrick S E et al 1992 Sequential changes in histological pattern and extracellular matrix deposition during the healing of chronic venous ulcers. American Journal of Pathology 141(5): 1085–1095

Hobbs J 1993 Varicose veins. In: Wolfe J (ed) ABC of vascular diseases. BMJ Publications, London

Hume M, Sevett S, Thomas D P 1970 Venous thrombosis and pulmonary embolism. Harvard University Press, Cambridge, Mass.

Kumar P J, Clark M L 1989 Clinical medicine. Baillière Tindall, London

Leitschuh M et al 1987 Vascular changes in hypertension. Medical Clinics of N America 71: 827–839

Muldoon M F et al 1990 Lowering cholesterol concentration and mortality, a qualitative review of primary prevention trials. British Medical Journal 301: 309–314

Robbs J 1990 An extension of the classification of Takayasu's disease and the management of inflammatory aneurysms in Japan. In: Greenhalgh R, Mannik (eds) The cause and management of aneurysms. Saunders, Philadelphia

Rosenow E C, Osmundson P J, Brown M I 1981 Pulmonary embolism. Mayo Clinic Proc 56: 161–178

Sooriakumaran S 1994 Prosthetic rehabilitation. Conference paper, Cardiff

Taylor P R 1993 Treating aortic aneurysms. In: Wolfe J (ed) ABC of vascular diseases. BMJ Publications, London

Thomas P R S et al 1988 White cell accumulation in dependent legs of patients with venous hypertension; a possible mechanism for topical changes in the skin. British Medical Journal 296: 1693–1695

Wolfe J 1993 ABC of vascular diseases. BMJ Publications, London

FURTHER READING

Schmid-Schorbein G W 1995 Activated leukocytes; a double edged sword. Wounds 7(5): 189–198

Ting M 1991 Wound healing and peripheral vascular disease. Critical Care Nursing Clinics of North America 3(3): 515

Prevention

Fish oils such as cod liver oil reduce platelet deposition, thrombosis and athero-sclerosis, because they contain two acids, elcosapentaenic acid (EPA) and docosa-hexaenoic acid (DHA), which are converted to form prostaglandins. These inhibit the synthesis of arachidonic acid which promotes platelet clumping (Laker 1991). EPA and DHA therefore have a similar physiological effect to prostacyclin (PGI_2).

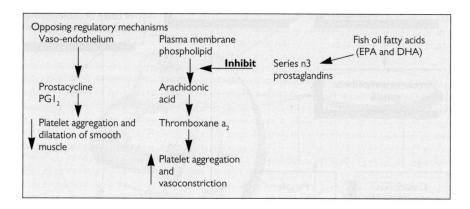

A balanced diet containing starch and fibre gives a satisfying feeling of fullness without providing too many calories; they help to prevent constipation and keep blood cholesterol levels down, so reducing peripheral vascular disease.

■ **BOX 3.1 Guideline for a healthy diet**

Suggest to patients that:

- food is there to be enjoyed in moderation
- variety in what we eat is healthy
- they should eat the right amount to be a healthy weight; this will vary for age, sex and level of activity
- they should try not to eat too much fat, sugar or salt
- the diet should provide plenty of vitamins and minerals—zinc, magnesium and vitamin C are all important ingredients in the process of healing
- keeping levels of alcohol within recommended limits pays.

Nutrition essential for wound healing includes:

- calories
- protein
- zinc
- copper
- magnesium
- iron
- vitamins A, B Group, C, D and E.

Fat intake can be reduced by:

- using semiskimmed milk
- buying lean cuts of meat
- removing skin from fish or chicken
- eating meat products, e.g. pies and sausages, in moderation only
- using alternative methods of cooking rather than frying
- draining off excess fat
- cutting down on crisps, cakes and chocolate
- buying low-fat dairy products (cheese, yogurt).

Figure 3.3 shows a woman presenting with xanthoma over the eyelids. This is due to the laying down of lipoids in the skin, indicative of high levels of serum cholesterol.

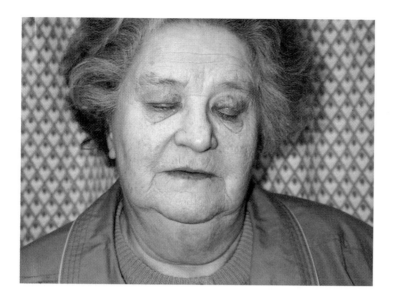

Fig. 3.3 A woman presenting with xanthoma over the eyelids.

Wound healing and diet

There is much evidence that poor nutrition delays wound healing. Peripheral vascular patients' wounds healed more slowly if they had low serum albumin and low transferrin (an enzyme associated with the absorption of iron). Protein malnutrition is also associated with non-healing ulcers, probably because of defective collagen synthesis.

The need for an adequate supply of glucose may increase dramatically where major wound healing is taking place. Fatty acids are required for the production of prostaglandins and prostacyclins.

Among the trace elements, *zinc*, which is found in meat, fish and nuts, is a co-factor for more than 200 enzymes which help manufacture protein, carbohydrate, fat and nucleic acids. *Copper* is necessary for collagen synthesis and is available in liver, fish, nuts and chocolate. Lack of *iron* causes reduced haemoglobin in the blood and consequently reduces the oxygen that is available to the wound. Iron is supplied by meat, liver and green vegetables.

Deficiency of *B vitamins* interferes with immunity, enzyme action and, like that of *vitamins C and A*, collagen synthesis; deficiencies may present as a non-healing wound or ulcer, or scurvy. *Vitamin E* is needed for the integrity of cell membranes.

Salt

Some believe that, in a bid to reduce blood pressure, a reduction in salt intake should be promoted.

Salt intake can be cut by:

- reducing the amount used in cooking
- reducing intake of salty snacks, e.g. crisps, salted nuts
- reducing intake of salted foods, e.g. bacon, cheese and shellfish in brine.

Alcohol

The proportion of people drinking more than the sensible limits of alcohol should be fewer than 1 in 6 in men and 1 in 18 in women. Current recommended safe levels for alcohol consumption are shown in Figure 3.4.

These levels are currently under review. However, Gazinao et al (1993) suggest that 'moderate alcohol intake increases the protection factors of HDL lipoproteins which reduces the risk of coronary heart disease'.

Men 28 units	**Women 21 units**

One unit is equal to half a pint of beer, a single measure of spirit or one small glass of wine.

Fig. 3.4 Current recommendations for safe weekly alcohol limits.

Reduction of obesity

Obesity can be defined as being more than 7 kilograms over the normal recommended weight for height (body mass index).

Obesity = more than 7 kg over normal recommended weight for height.

$$BMI = \frac{(body\ mass\ in\ kilograms)^2}{height\ in\ metres}$$

Normal values should be < 26 in women and < 27 in men.

Reduction in obesity will be achieved through positive psychological attitudes, attention to portion size and content, and exercise, supported by appropriate health promotion. The Department of Health's recommendations for a healthy, well-balanced diet are illustrated in Figure 3.5.

Physical exercise

Physical exercise promotes:

- strength, stamina, suppleness
- development of arterial collateral blood supply
- venous return,

Exercise builds strength, suppleness and stamina. It reduces the incidence of obesity, strengthens the heart and lungs through aerobic activity and adds strength to bones through weight-bearing exercise. It encourages the development of collateral circulations which, in the diseased limb, may be all-important in preventing ischaemia. Relaxation can also be achieved through exercise in the management of stress and insomnia.

In uncomplicated hypertension (i.e. hypertension devoid of symptoms or signs) regular moderate exercise is beneficial. However, whilst this group should be encouraged to improve and maintain their fitness, caution is required and strenuous isometric or dynamic exercise should be avoided in order to reduce the risk of myocardial infarction (Sannerstedt 1987). Exercise also increases HDL levels in the plasma, so helping to protect against peripheral vascular disease (Curfman 1993).

Table 3.1 shows the effect of various exercise activities on strength, stamina and suppleness.

The fact that exercise pre-operatively improves strength is also of use in the postoperative situation, especially for amputees. It is widely held that patients who are fit pre-operatively do better postoperatively.

Further, improved tone of muscles and increased exercise prevent venous pooling by increasing venous return.

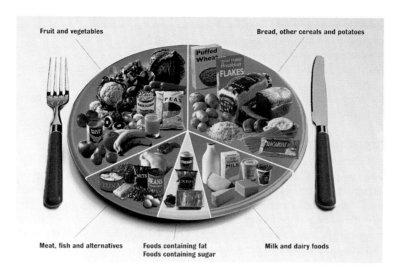

Fig. 3.5 The proportions of different types of foods that make up a healthy diet. (Reproduced with kind permission from the Health Education Authority.)

Table 3.1 The effect of various exercise activities on stamina, suppleness and strength

Activities	Stamina	Suppleness	Strength
Badminton	2	3	2
Climbing stairs	0	1	2
Cricket	1	2	1
Cycling (hard)	4	2	3
Dancing (ballroom)	1	3	1
Dancing (disco)	3	4	1
Gardening (digging)	3	2	4
Football	3	3	3
Golf	1	2	1
Hill walking	3	1	2
Housework	1	2	1
Jogging	4	2	2
Mowing the lawn	2	1	3
Squash	3	2	2
Swimming	4	4	4
Tennis	2	3	2
Walking (briskly)	3	2	1
Weightlifting	1	1	4
Yoga	1	4	1

1 = No real effect   2 = Beneficial effect   3 = Very good effect   4 = Excellent effect

As a result of the recommendations made, physical exercise is now a compulsory part of the National Curriculum for all children aged 5–16. It is hoped that good habits relating to physical exercise will be instilled from an early age, so reducing the incidence of disease as this generation becomes older. Shinton demonstrated that 'appreciable protection from stroke in later life is conferred by vigorous exercise in early adulthood. This increased level of exercise should, if possible, be continued throughout life to maintain the protective effect' (Shinton 1993).

Several bodies, such as the National Sports Council, local councils, the Departments of Health and Education and employers, are now running initiatives to promote physical fitness for people of all ages.

Warning Always advise patients to warm up first before sudden bursts of physical activity, as failure to do so may increase the risk of cardiac strain.

Patients need to be advised to stop the activities if they feel any pain or dizziness, or are unwell.

Patient tolerance to exercise programmes

For the patient with mild peripheral vascular disease experiencing intermittent claudication, compliance and benefits brought about through the opening up of collateral blood vessels are probably greater than for the patient with moderate or severe vascular disease. For the latter patient, a regime of passive leg exercises, such as pumping the foot/calf muscle pumps through gentle movement of the leg, may be the limit of his or her capabilities, at least until surgical intervention has reduced the symptoms of pain.

Patients need to choose programmes of exercise which:

- they enjoy
- can be done on a regular basis, e.g. walking, swimming three times a week
- fit easily into the daily routine
- are within their individual capabilities.

Regular vigorous exercise for 20 minutes, three times a week, is recommended. Recent studies have shown that brisk walking at the above frequency and duration can reduce the risk of peripheral vascular disease (Ernst 1991).

Exercise and calorie consumption

Figure 3.6 shows the time required to burn up 100 calories of energy with various forms of exercise.

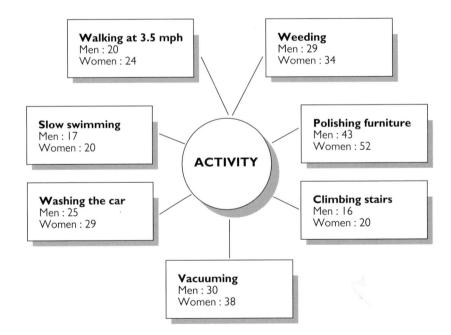

Fig. 3.6 The time required (in minutes) to burn up 100 calories of energy with various forms of exercise.

Care of the diabetic foot/amputation

In an attempt to reduce the number of amputations both for diabetes and arterial disease, the patient will need to understand clearly the significance of the following:

• Wearing appropriate shoes and protecting feet from trauma and damage due to pressure, resulting in callus formation.

• Taking care in cutting toenails, especially where diabetic neuropathy and ischaemia exist. Referral to a chiropodist should be considered to prevent toenails being cut too short, so increasing the risk of damage to tissues through trauma.

• Inspecting the feet daily, checking for callus formation, ulceration, infection or trauma. Immediate medical referral should be made if these are found to be present.

• Keeping the feet clean and dry. This will help to reduce the risk of infection. If skin becomes dehydrated there is an increased risk of cracks and tissue breakdown, resulting in ulceration. The use of barrier creams will reduce this risk. It is recognized that creams containing lanolin are more likely to cause allergic responses, and these should therefore be avoided.

• Not smoking and appropriate management of diet and exercise. These will assist in slowing the process of atherosclerosis.

Stress

A degree of pressure in life is said to be beneficial and increases efficiency of performance. However, pressure in excess of ability to cope generates stress. This is the result of continuously high levels of anxiety. The body's natural response to anxiety is to release adrenaline, so preparing the body for action—'fight or flight'. This increases the heart rate and the response of the nervous system, and, in the liver, steps up the release of glucose, cholesterol and fatty acids into the circulation. The body becomes 'stressed'. This results in hypertension and, over a longer period of time, promotes atherosclerosis and a reduction in the efficiency of the immune system.

Symptoms of stress are outlined in Figure 3.7.

Suggested steps to cope with stress

• if possible, identify what is causing the stress
• organize effective use of time
• take regular exercise, especially rhythmic exercise, e.g. walking, swimming
• avoid excessive consumption of alcohol, smoking and compulsive eating

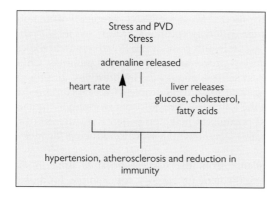

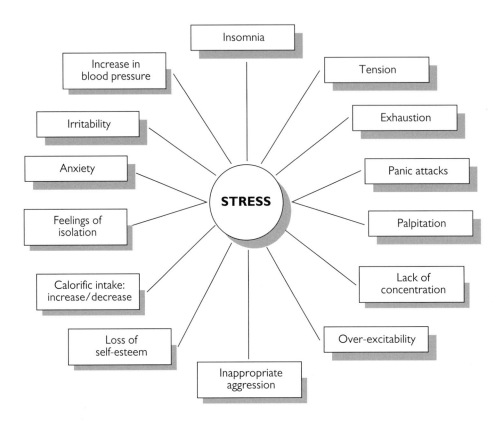

Fig. 3.7 Symptoms of stress.

- learn relaxation techniques, e.g. listening to music, yoga, deep controlled breathing.

Reduction of stress will help in the prevention of vascular disease. The need for surgery may place patients and their families under immense stress, and the practitioner needs to recognize this and provide support.

THE CHALLENGE TO THE PROFESSION

As a profession we are faced with quite a challenge in assisting those people we care for to achieve the *Health of the Nation* targets. Fortunately information and resources, usually provided by voluntary groups and local health promotion units, are available for use in health promotion. Practitioners in the community are ideally placed to develop preventative disease programmes. Children are receiving more information in schools about healthy lifestyles, and the nation is becoming more aware of the need to address problems which could reduce the quality and quantity of life in the long term. Practitioners working in the secondary care sector are also in a good position to heighten patients' awareness of risk factors as they are discharged from hospital, with a view to reducing the incidence of future disease.

Supporting patients from the earliest possible time in making changes in lifestyle may reduce the need for surgery, for example, for those with claudication.

It will also speed up their recovery following surgery. If new patterns of behaviour can be maintained, there may be an overall improvement in quality of life.

Presentation of information

Effective communication is an essential element of health promotion. Body language, eye contact, tone, clarity, structure and content of material presented all need to be considered (Beaver 1986).

In presenting information, one needs to respect the values and preferences of the individuals being supported. Only if they want change themselves will this be brought about. Their desire for change is more likely to increase if they have a sound knowledge base from which to make decisions (Becker et al 1980). Where they are able to participate actively, health promotion is more effective. They also need to have trust in the person supporting them. That person must be able to listen, understand and show compassion, while helping the patient to set realistic goals at the outset and to maintain the motivation to change behaviour patterns (Bandura 1977, Gange 1985, Kramer 1972, Maslow 1971, Rogers 1951, 1983).

The presentation and readability of literature used to reinforce information given to people needs also to be carefully considered. The Flesch readability scale measures the ease with which literature can be read.

Information presented in small chunks, with short sentences and paragraphs, colour or cartoons with short captions to captivate the audience, and changes in print to highlight new sections or important words will all aid the effectiveness of the resource as a useful health-promotion tool. People are more likely to remember something if the aural information is supported by a visual resource which is jargon-free.

Learners remember

- 20% of what they hear
- 30% of what they see
- 50% of what they see and hear
- 70% of what they say
- 90% of what they say and do (Green & Faden 1977).

Factors conducive to learning are outlined in Figure 3.8.

> Health promotion material needs to be:
> - eye-catching
> - easy to read
> - jargon-free
> - memorable.

Guidelines for patients' pre-admission for vascular surgery and on discharge

Where patients are to be admitted from a waiting list for surgery, the time between deciding that surgery is appropriate and admission can be used fruitfully in health promotion, so reducing the risk of postoperative complications associated with smoking, obesity and poor mobility. The following guidelines are relevant to both the pre-admission period and the period after discharge from the acute setting.

> Successful pre-operative health promotion will help to reduce postoperative morbidity and mortality.

Smoking

Where time allows, it is important to encourage the patient to stop smoking prior to admission. This will reduce the number of postoperative chest infections and further reduce ongoing risks from increasing atherosclerotic plaque formation. Even stopping smoking 12 hours before the operation will reduce the risks associated with anaesthetic, as carbon monoxide levels are reduced.

Postoperatively, the contribution of smoking to arterial disease needs to be explained to the patient if he or she is to understand why continuing to smoke will increase the risk of disease and the need for further surgery. *Nicotine impregnated patches and chewing gum*, which are now available from chemists, can help patients to stop smoking.

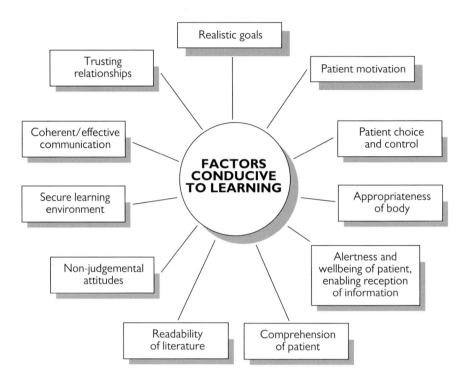

Fig. 3.8 Factors conducive to learning.

Diet

If the patient is overweight, a well-balanced reducing diet should be encouraged, containing proteins, vitamins A, B group, C and D, zinc and magnesium, to promote healing. Some polyunsaturated fat is beneficial, providing this does not exceed the recommended total of 20% of the daily intake of energy. High fibre will also be beneficial in preventing constipation.

Any special diet will need to be catered for, and the support of a dietician should be called on as needed.

Alcohol

The patient should stay within recommended limits for alcohol intake, as discussed previously.

Exercise

Exercise is important in helping patients retain suppleness of joints and in the development of collateral blood circulation. Tightening the buttocks and muscles of the leg will help prevent DVT. Exercises to strengthen the arms will improve the patient's mobility after the operation. Giving patients something positive to do will make them feel that they are helping themselves, and therefore help them to develop a positive attitude to their recovery. Gaining freedom of movement will also reduce pressure necrosis and the development of pressure sores, as will placing a monkey pole over the bed and encouraging the patient to periodically lift his or her buttocks off the bed. This procedure will also help to strengthen arms. Enhanced mobility, again, will cut down the risk of chest infections.

Relaxation

Stress is a factor in the hardening of the arteries, and a high degree of anxiety will increase stress. This can greatly be reduced if the patient learns to relax. Anxiety regarding surgery can be reduced by giving sufficient information to patients before and after admission in order to help them prepare themselves.

Sleep

A good night's sleep will help the general well-being of patients. Sedation or alternative therapies used in a controlled way can help to promote sound sleep in order that patients do not become exhausted. They will be better able to recover from surgery if they are not overtired.

On discharge from hospital as an outpatient

Health promotion to encourage a healthy lifestyle needs to be continued after discharge, as arterial disease is not usually confined to one segment of the body.

Medication

Following some arterial procedures—e.g. aortic aneurysm repair, arterial bypass reconstruction surgery and carotid endarterectomy—some centres may prescribe daily aspirin to reduce the risk of thrombus formation, which is high in such cases because of the possibility of generalized arterial disease. Repeat prescriptions for aspirin and any other necessary medication will need to be obtained from the patient's general practitioner, who will have been informed of his or her discharge by the medical team.

Returning to work

Where this is applicable, patients will need to be individually advised by the medical staff. Consideration will need to be given to the patient's physical status, type of surgery undertaken and what is involved in their work, e.g. heavy lifting or driving.

Working at home

The above principles should be applied even if patients are retired. They should be encouraged to rest and not lift anything heavier than their dinner tray for 2–3 weeks. It may take 3–6 months before they are able to achieve the same level of activity that they enjoyed pre-operatively. Advising patients of this will help to ensure that expectations are realistic.

Exercise

Initially, during the first 3–4 weeks, gentle exercise should be encouraged—for example, if it is physically possible a daily walk in the fresh air is recommended, combined with rest. Gradually strength will be regained and patients will increase their exercise tolerance on an individual basis. Exercises such as swimming, jogging or racket sports should not be resumed for at least 4–6 weeks—one should remember that the tissues and muscles inside need to heal and become strong first.

Driving

Patients must be able to perform an emergency stop. They should allow a minimum of 4 weeks after abdominal and lower limb surgery before driving, as this puts quite a strain on the stomach and leg muscles. It is advisable to wait at least 2 more weeks before driving long distances. Most insurance companies suggest that patients should check with their doctor before recommencing.

Bathing

Once the wound is dry, and even before the stitches are removed, it is acceptable for the patient to bath or shower.

The wound

Arrangements will need to be made with the community nurse for ongoing wound care and removal of skin closures on the appropriate postoperative day. Should the patient notice any abnormal discharge, inflammation or pain, they should not hesitate to seek medical advice.

Sexual activity

There is no restriction on patients enjoying a normal sex life by 2 or 3 weeks after discharge, providing they feel happy about doing so. They should be advised to be gentle at first, as they would when recommencing any other form of physical activity. Impotence can present as a complication of aneurysmal and ileac surgery, depending on the surgical technique used. Should this arise their consultant or general practitioner can make a referral, if necessary, to an erectile dysfunction specialist for advice and counselling. Through self-administration of drugs or the use of penile supports an erection may be achieved and normal sexual activity maintained.

Home support

Evaluation of patients' need for home support will have begun on admission to hospital and will need implementation on discharge. An assessment of needs should also be made if they are being cared for in the community. If it is considered appropriate by the patient and the nursing staff, support will be arranged at home (e.g. meals on wheels, home help) until he or she feels able to cope alone.

Meeting the challenge of health promotion

In both the primary and secondary care sectors, evaluating the effectiveness of health promotion should become the norm in today's climate of clinical audit, as we measure effectiveness of care against set standards or outcomes. Using the recommendations in the *Health of the Nation* document when deciding outcomes will help to ensure that the targets set for the year 2000 are maintained.

REFERENCES

Bandura A 1977 Social learning theory. Prentice-Hall, Englewood Cliffs, N J
Beaver B 1986 Health education and the patient with peripheral vascular disease. Nursing Clinics of North America 21(2): 265–272
Becker M et al 1980 Strategies for changing patient compliance. Journal of Community Health 6: 113–135
Curfman G D 1993 New England Journal of Medicine 329(23): 1730–1731
Department of Health 1991 Health of the nation. HMSO, London
Ernst E 1991 Peripheral vascular disease: benefits of exercise. Sports Medicine 12(3): 149–151
Ewles L, Simnett I 1995 Promoting health: a practical guide, 3rd edn. Scutari, London
Fawcett Hennessy A 1987 Recent advances in nursing. Professional Nurse 21: 170–194
Gange J 1985 The conditions of learning and theory of instruction. Holt, Rinehart & Winston, New York
Gaziano J M et al 1993 Alcohol HDL levels and risk of myocardial infarction. New England Journal of Medicine 329(25): 1829–1833

Green S, Faden R 1977 Potential effects on the patient. Drug Information Journal 3: 645–705
Hobbs J 1993 In: Wolfe J (ed) ABC of vascular diseases. BMJ Publications, London
Kramer M 1972 The concept of modelling as a teaching strategy. Nursing Forum 11: 50–69
Laker M, Alberti K 1991 Fish oils: fact or fantasy. Hospital Update 17(4): 283–290
MacSweeney S T R et al 1994 Smoking and growth rate of small abdominal aortic
    aneurysms. Lancet 344: 651–652
Maslow A 1971 The farther reaches of human nature. Penguin, Harmondsworth
Rogers C 1951 Client centred therapy. Houghton Mifflin, Boston
Rogers C 1983 Freedom to learn for the 80s. Merrill, Ohio
Sannerstedt R 1993 Hypertension. In: Skinner J S (ed) 1993 Exercise testing and exercise
    prescription for special cases. Theoretical basis and clinical application. Febiger,
    Philadelphia
Shinton R 1993 Lifelong exercise and stroke reduction. British Medical Journal 307(6898):
    231–234
Ralph C 1990 A strategy for nursing: the UKCC view. Nursing Standard 5(6 Suppl): 7–10
Which? 1993 Which? way to health. April Which?, London
West Midlands Regional Health Authority Directorate of Nursing and Quality 1992 Health
    Promotion in Nursing—the way to the future. Unpublished

FURTHER READING

Blackburn C 1994 Low income inequality and health promotion. Nursing Times 90(39):
    42–43
Bunton R (ed) 1991 Health promotion disciplines diversity. Routledge, London
Cox B D 1993 The health and lifestyle survey. Dartmouth Publishing, London
Dengel D et al 1994 Comparable effects of diet and exercise on body composition and
    lipoproteins in older men. Medicine and Science in Sports and Exercise 26(11): 1307–1315
Dines A (ed) 1994 Health promotion concepts and practice. Blackwell, Oxford
Doll R et al 1994 Mortality in relation to smoking: 40 years' observation in male British
    doctors. British Medical Journal 309(6959): 901–911
Edelman C L 1994 Health promotion throughout the lifespan, 3rd edn. Mosby, London
Grace M L et al 1994 Nutritional education for patients with peripheral vascular disease.
    Journal of Health Education 25(3): 142–146
Halliwell B 1993 Free radicals and vascular disease: how much do we know? British Medical
    Journal 307(6909): 885–886
Health Education 1993 Health promotion and the reforms in primary health. Health
    Education Authority, London
Holmes S 1994 Nutrition and older people—A matter for concern. Nursing Times 90(42):
    31–33
Mansell P 1991 Garlic: effects on serum lipids, blood pressure, coagulation, platelet
    aggregation, and vasodilatation. British Medical Journal 303(6799): 379–380
Marshall W 1994 Lipid lowering: the drugs and diet. Practice Nursing 5(17): 14–16
McSweeney et al 1994 Smoking and the growth rate of small abdominal aortic aneurysms.
    Lancet 344: 651
Murray R B, Zentner J P 1988 Nursing concepts for health promotion, 3rd edn. Prentice-Hall,
    Englewood Cliffs, N J
Paffenbarger Jr R S et al 1993 Life style changes and mortality in men. New England Journal
    of Medicine 328(8): 538–545
Pedoe H T 1994–95 Cardiovascular benefits of quitting smoking. Journal of Smoking-related
    Disorders Supp 1: 55–59
Schatz M 1994 Stressed out? Physician and Sports Medicine 22(11): 87–88
Stamford B 1994 Staying fit as you age. Physician and Sports Medicine 22(10): 111–112
Tolley K 1993 Health promotion: how to measure cost-effectiveness. Health Education
    Authority, London
Walkabout to Health 1994 A pilot promotion: effectiveness and cost implications. Journal of
    the Institute of Health and Education 32(3): 76–80
Webb P 1993 Health promotion and patient education. Chapman & Hall, London
Welsh Office 1990 Health for all in Wales strategies for action. HMSO, London
Wilson-Barnett J 1993 Research in health promotion and nursing. Macmillan, London

Understanding pain and its management

CHAPTER 4

PERCEPTION OF PAIN

What is pain? Why does the amputee experience phantom limb pain? Pain is subjective, but from research we know that it originates objectively through proven mechanisms. Merskey (1964) states that 'Pain is an unpleasant experience which we primarily associate with tissue damage, or describe in terms of tissue, damage or both'.

Ischaemia, along with the build-up of endorphins and waste metabolites would all contribute to an increase of pain if there is insufficient perfusion of oxygenated blood. The nerve endings cannot tolerate ischaemia as well as the skin can. Moderate pain may be demonstrated by a rise in blood pressure. If the pain is severe blood pressure may drop, with a corresponding increase in pulse rate. Referred pain is an embryological phenomenon based on the fact that two distant structures arose originally from the same primitive area, for example the heart and the inner aspect of the left arm (angina).

Pain may be considered as an exaggeration of normal sensory signals and be positively utilized to promote a response which will alleviate or prevent further damage, by enforcing rest to promote healing. The diabetic with sensory neuropathy in the feet may incur severe trauma which could not be tolerated by other individuals normally responsive to pain.

Various ideas about the mechanism of the perception of pain have evolved. The idea of pain as a specific sensation carried in pain pathways from the peripheral nerves to the brain is outmoded. It was previously assumed that nerve fibres relayed the sensation directly to the thalamus and that, when the signals were sufficiently intense, pain was felt.

As pain can present as different sensations—for example, burning, a sharpness, a dull ache—it has been suggested that a whole pattern of nervous impulses are evoked in response to tissue damage. The complex impulses travel with sensory impulses, and only when the brain decodes the pattern and intensity is pain experienced.

Important among this pattern of impulses are two pathways:

• A force injuring the skin (for example) activates so-called mechanosensitive nociceptors and the impulse travels up fast (small, myelinated) fibres to the thalamus and thence to the cortex. These fibres tend to be non-branching, so the eventual experience is very specific and localized.

• At the same time, in contrast, other receptors, polymodal nociceptors, send a wide variety of stimuli to the brain in larger, unmyelinated slow fibres. These synapse and branch several times en route and eventually produce a vague ache. It is thought that it is these fibres which communicate with the hypothalamus and other structures to produce an emotional response to pain (Rutishauser 1994).

Because such a wide variety of sensory impulses are activated as 'pain', it is not surprising that in some circumstances particular nerve fibres predominate. So it is that paraesthesiae can occur, particularly when sensation is gradually returning to a numb limb.

In 1965 it was suggested that in the dorsal section of the spinal cord there are cells which modulate the transmission of the impulses from the periphery, allowing or disallowing impulses through a 'gate' (Melzach & Wall 1965). It was proposed that the control of these cells comes from the higher centres. The aim was to explain why it is that the perception of pain intensity depends on such higher 'influences' as personality, fear, experience and memory, and may be susceptible to counselling, hypnosis or yoga. The modulating cells in the spinal cord have been said to 'edit' the impulses (Youngson 1992).

Conversely, relatively minor impulses can be exaggerated by the modulating cells to become interpreted as pain. The suggestion is that the brain becomes sensitized to pain impulses, so that for a while they are exaggerated. The brain effectively learns that pain is present and memorizes it. At a cellular level, a number of protein molecules which are implicated in the discernment of pain have been identified—for example, NMDA (N-methyl d-aspartate) receptor protein. This has a relevance to the control of surgical and phantom pain, in that if these agents are not 'switched on' in the first place, the intensity and persistence of the pain will be less.

The original pain impulses need to be blocked before they reach these spinal receptors. A number of techniques attempt to do this.

> Gate theory of pain
>
> Pain impulses from the periphery to the brain face a 'gate' which is either open or closed and which is controlled by higher centres.

• *Transcutaneous electrical nerve stimulation.* The gate theory helps to explain why fast-conducting nerve fibres which are responsive to touch and mild mechanical stimulation (as may be found with a transcutaneous electrical nerve stimulation machine) travel alongside the slow-conducting, smaller pain-transmitting nerve fibres into the spinal cord. On arrival in the brain stem, the fast stimulus blocks the slower one, and hence the messages of pain are blocked out.

• *Local regional anaesthetic.* Patients receiving local nerve blocks for operations require less postoperative analgesia that those who have undergone a general anaesthetic (Youngson 1992). Receptors to morphine have been identified in the spinal cord. Indeed, morphine-like substances which may naturally diminish pain have been identified in vivo. These 'endogenous opioids' include endorphins, encephalins and dymorphin.

If morphine is injected close to the spine, but outside the dura mater (i.e. epidural block), enough diffuses through to the receptors to produce a profound analgesia at a much lower dosage than a systemic dose of morphine. However, the side-effects of intrathecal morphine can be fatal, as occasionally it can travel in the cerebrospinal fluid to the brain where it exerts a dramatic inhibitory effect on respiration, equivalent to that caused by a massive overdose.

If a combination of a synthetic opioid such as fentanyl, which is more lipid-soluble, and local anaesthetic is used, the analgesic effect is achieved by a lower dose with fewer side-effects.

Postoperative discomfort is kept to a minimum by the use of patient-controlled analgesia (PCA) or by a continuous epidural infusion of analgesics (Thomas 1995). After the first 48 hours pain is usually found to be minimal, and mild oral analgesics are sufficient to maintain control.

• *Patient-controlled analgesia* allows a regulated infusion of analgesic. This is delivered at the command of the patients. It puts them physically in control so that they do not have to wait for analgesia to be administered by nursing staff and can receive a rapid response to the sensation of pain before endorphins have been allowed to build up. It has been found that, with this method, patients require less opioid than if it is administered in the traditional way.

It is correct to state that it is easier to keep a patient comfortable than to relieve agony. A patient who awakens free from pain can be kept comfortable more easily. According to Youngson (1992), 'Patients for gall-bladder surgery who are given epidural anaesthesia have been shown to recover and leave hospital two days earlier than those who have conventional anaesthetics'.

PCAs have been found to be safe in that the dose administered is self-limiting owing to the state of consciousness of the patient and an equipment lock-out facility which operates when the maximum dose for a set period of time has been received.

As opioids may cause nausea, anti-emetics are often prescribed with them. There has been debate as to whether opioids and anti-emetics are stable when mixed in one syringe for administration via a PCA. However, Williams et al (1992) have shown that a combination of morphine and droperidol is stable for up to 14 days. Should there be any reason for concern, the addition of a filter between the syringe and percutaneous cannula could provide a safety barrier should crystallization have occurred.

• *Non-steroidal anti-inflammatory drugs (NSAIDs)*. Tissue damage triggers an inflammatory response, and inflammatory agents provoke pain. Pre-operative administration of NSAIDs reduces postoperative consumption of analgesics.

• *NMDA receptor blockers* are currently being researched.

• *Simple interventions* will also prove invaluable, such as suggesting to patients that they should inform nursing staff if they are not comfortable. Many patients will not ask because they do not wish to 'bother the nurse' or simply because they do not realize they can ask for analgesia. Boore (1994) noted that informing patients about their situation will reduce pain, not simply because they understand what is happening to them, but rather because they know they can ask for analgesics.

A bed cradle may be helpful in reducing the pressure of the bed linen.

• *Alternative therapies*. Many nurses today are taking an interest in, and training in, alternative therapies which can have a positive effect on the patient's recovery through a reduction in anxiety. Music therapy, relaxation, reflexology, massage, aromatherapy and the sense of touch can offer a great sense of comfort when used appropriately. This fact corroborates the gate theory in pain management. The mere presence of another person, such as a relative or close friend, can provide comfort, without the necessity to talk.

Massage combines the benefits of many of these therapies. Correctly applied relaxation massage can help reduce anxiety and stress, induce sleep and assist in the relief of chronic pain as the patient relaxes and takes the tension out of the muscles. It is a useful way of demonstrating caring. Massage enhances arterial and venous blood flow and lymphatic drainage, so improving diffusion of nutrients and oxygen to tissues (Evans 1994).

In nursing today there is less physical contact with patients. Gone are the times when nurses did 'back rounds', as research has demonstrated the dangers of friction caused by rubbing the skin with talcum powder. However, there was much to be said for the comfort given to patients simply by turning pillows and massaging aching backs.

Touch could be construed as an invasion of a person's privacy and physical space, and this is something the nurse needs to be aware of in approaching patients. In 1982 Quinn objectively tested the hypothesis that touch therapy has a positive effect on patients, comparing subjects treated with compassionate touch with a sample for whom touch was minimized, and demonstrated that there was a decrease in anxiety scores in subjects treated with real touch. This supports the work performed by Keller, Heidt and Krieger (Sayre-Adams 1994).

Music therapy uses the medium of music to facilitate and enhance relaxation, particularly if it is calming music with long note durations, gently flowing rhythmic patterns, a slow tempo and soft dynamics. Instruments such as the flute, harp, piano and pan pipes are ideal in providing music therapy. Alternatively, patients may simply enjoy losing themselves in the music of their favourite artist.

PCA

• puts the patient in control
• is safe
• gives immediate relief
• saves nursing time
• reduces analgesic requirement
• reduces postoperative complications, e.g. DVT and chest infections.

Patients need to know:

• how to take analgesics
• when to take analgesics
• with what frequency to take analgesics
• that they should inform carers if analgesia is not effective.

Alternative therapies to analgesic medication:

• relaxation
• music
• aromatherapy
• massage
• real touch
• acupuncture
• yoga
• meditation,

Humour is a unique, 'high touch' human medium which can indicate a personal and caring approach and play a role in reducing stress (Hillman 1994).

• *A multidisciplinary* approach to pain management has been shown to be beneficial, leading to changes in nursing and medical practice and the production of joint pain assessment instruments. More-effective techniques and medication for pain control then become possible.

MONITORING PAIN

> Monitoring pain using an effective tool will enhance pain control.

A number of studies have suggested that since pain is so subjective and individual to the person experiencing it, the most appropriate method of pain determination is a 'pain thermometer' numerical rating scale of 1 to 10. Descriptive scales have not proved to be as effective in clinical trials (Downie et al 1978, Haywood 1994, Jones 1988, Scott 1992).

DEALING WITH PAIN IN THE NON-SURGICAL SETTING: A GUIDE FOR THE SELECTION OF APPROPRIATE ANALGESIA

Variations are bound to exist from centre to centre as to an exact regime for the prescription of opiates, but the following represents a ladder of analgesic choice (Fig. 4.1).

Once opiates have been started they should be increased as required, using morphine sulphate solution or the equivalent every 4 hours:

5 mg ⟶ 10 mg ⟶ 15 mg ⟶ 20 mg ⟶ 30 mg

and so on, with no upper limit if there are no intolerable side-effects.

Fig. 4.1 'Ladder' of choice for different levels of pain relief.

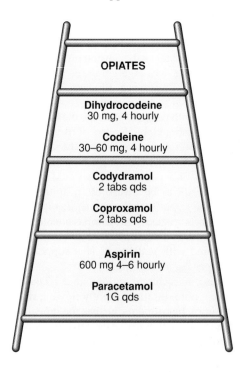

OPIATES

Dihydrocodeine
30 mg, 4 hourly

Codeine
30–60 mg, 4 hourly

Codydramol
2 tabs qds

Coproxamol
2 tabs qds

Aspirin
600 mg 4–6 hourly

Paracetamol
1G qds

Once the dose is stable the medication may be converted to sustained release tablets. Each twice-daily dose is calculated by totalling the dose given in 24 hours and dividing by 2, the first dose being given 4 hours after the last dose of solution.

Fear of addiction to opioids when they are required to control severe pain has been proved to be unfounded (Ferrell 1992).

Adjuvants that may be necessary with opiates include anti-emetics and laxatives. For breakthrough pain, other medication may be used for additional analgesic effect, for example:

- Dexamethasone for nerve compression
- Amitriptyline or carbamazepine for stabbing or neuropathic pain.

REFERENCES

Boore J 1994 Prescription for recovery. Scutari, London

Downie W et al 1978 Studies with pain rating scales. Ann Rhum Dis: 37(4): 378–381

Evans J 1994 Relaxation massage in nursing practice. Unpublished

Ferrell B 1992 Pain and addiction: an urgent need for change in nursing education. Journal of Pain and Symptom Management 7(2): 117–123

Haywood J 1994 Information—a prescription against pain. Scutari, London

Hillman S 1994 The healing power of humour at work. Nursing Standard 8(42): 31–34

Jones C 1988 Pain assessment. Surg Nurse 1(7): 5–8

Melzack R, Wall P D 1965 Pain mechanisms; a new theory. Science 150: 971–975

Merskey H 1964 An investigation of pain in psychological illness. DN thesis, Oxford

Quinn J 1989 Future direction for therapeutic touch research. Journal of Holistic Nursing 7(1): 19–25

Rutishauser S 1994 Physiology and anatomy: a basis for nursing and health care. Churchill Livingstone, Edinburgh

Sayre-Adams J 1994 Therapeutic touch: a nursing function. Nursing Standard 8(17): 25–28

Scott I 1992 Nurses' attitudes to pain control and the use of pain assessment scales. British Journal of Nursing 2(1): 11–15

Thomas N 1995 Patient controlled analgesia. Nursing Standard 35: 31–37

Williams O A 1992 Stability of morphine and droperidol, separately and combined for use as an infusion. Hosp Pharm Pract 2(9): 545–549

Youngson R 1992 Pathways to pain control. New Scientist 21st March: 24–27

FURTHER READING

Balfour S E 1989 Will I be in pain? Patients' and nurses' attitudes to pain after abdominal surgery. Prof Nurse 5(1): 28–33

Cohen P L 1980 Post surgical pain relief: patient status and nurses' medication choices. Pain 9: 266–274

Chien B B et al 1991 An extensive experience with postoperative pain relief using postoperative fentanyl infusion. Archives of Surgery 126(6): 692–694

Dahl J B et al 1992 Differential analgesic effects of low dose epidural morphine and morphine/bupivacaine at rest and during mobilisation after major abdominal surgery. Anaesthesia and Analgesia 1974(3): 362–365

Davis P S 1988 Changing nursing practice for more effective control of postoperative pain through a staff initiated educational programme. Nurse Education Today 6(8): 325–331

Gooch J 1989 Who should manage pain: patient or nurse? Prof Nurse 4(6): 295–296

Keeney S A 1993 Nursing care of the post operative patient receiving epidural analgesia. Nursing 2(3): 191–196

Latham J 1994 Simple analgesics—choosing with care. RCN Nursing Update. Nursing Standard 9(3): 1–13

Lesson L 1985 Pain and the post-operative patient. Nursing 2: 289–290

Melzach R 1975 The McGill pain questionnaire. Major properties and scoring methods. Pain 1(3): 277–299

Pediani R 1994 Recent developments in the control of surgical wound pain. Journal of Wound Care 3(8): 394–396

Raiman J 1986 Towards understanding pain and planning for relief. Use of the London Hospital Pain Observation Chart. Nursing 3(1): 411–422

Ready L B 1991 Postoperative epidural morphine is safe on surgical wards. Anaesthesiology 1975(3): 452–456

Ryder E 1991 All about patient controlled analgesia. Journal of Intravenous Nursing 14(6): 371–382

Soafer B 1983 Pain relief. The core of nursing practice. Nursing Times 29(46): 38–42

Vandenbosh T M 1988 How to use a pain flow sheet effectively. Nursing 18(8): 50–51

Assessment

Assessment of the vascular patient

This chapter is a window into assessments which may be performed to aid a differential diagnosis and to determine the feasibility of surgery and to ensure that vascular patients are adequately prepared prior to interventions. It is essential to monitor the physical status of the patient during hospitalization and, after the operation, to make an ongoing assessment of the patient's well-being, so that planned care can be sensitive and relevant to individual needs. Objective investigations can serve either to supply new data or to quantify what has already been learnt from the history and examination. The advent of modern technology permits surgical intervention to be more accurate and the results to be more predictable.

As arterial disease is rarely confined to one part of the body, patients need to be assessed fully for coexisting disease in all systems of the body.

In accordance with rule 18, nurses registered on Part 1 of the professional register need to be able to *assess*, plan, implement and evaluate care.

> Nurses have a responsibility to assess, plan, implement and evaluate.

Demographic details

The financial status of a patient may make a difference to his or her ability to comply with treatment. For example, the father who has three dependent children and an elderly relative to care for is not going to be able to take as much bed rest as the patient who is retired, single and able to afford support in the home, even if this is the appropriate care.

Past medical history

It is important in bringing to light related diseases, as discussed in Chapter 2.

Activities of daily living

Vascular patients may experience interference with activities of daily living, such as mobility, sleep and nutrition due to pain. The patient's ability to communicate and understand should be acknowledged so that *responsive management* can be implemented, ensuring that the patient's needs are met.

Assessment of risk factors

This will include smoking, obesity, poor nutrition, excessive use of alcohol and drugs, poor social supports, previous history of DVT and known coexisting disease (e.g. diabetes, hypertension, coronary heart disease, asthma or chronic obstructive airways disease).

Current medication

Patients' medication is a good indicator of any known medical conditions, e.g. hypertension, cardiac disorders or diabetes. The level of analgesia required to control pain may be an indicator as to the severity of ischaemia. It needs to be recognised that in the ischaemic patient beta-blockers may increase vasoconstriction and any previous reactions or contraindications to medication observed.

Allergies

Identifying and *recording* any medications, wound care products and other allergens will help to ensure *communication* with other health care professionals in order that safe practice is maintained.

Pain

The cause, position, intensity and type of sensation experienced plus the effectiveness of analgesia must be determined. Pain may be associated with:

- Pressure sores.
- Abdominal obstruction (occasionally) following aortic surgery.
- Flatulence or indigestion.
- Arthritis: many vascular patients will be in the elderly age group and present with coexisting conditions such as arthritis.
- Venous claudication, when pain is described as a bursting sensation, or a dull ache and heaviness of the legs. This is often the result of prolonged standing and is relieved by leg elevation.
- Arterial ischaemia, presenting as claudication or rest pain. Claudication pain is often described as cramp-like or sharp pain. This may be brought on by walking and relieved by resting. Also, pain which is felt in the foot, calf or buttocks at night and which is relieved by hanging the legs out of the bed may be indicative of ischaemia. This is expanded on in Chapters 8 and 9.

Pressure sore risk assessment

Arterial patients may well present with a high risk score, even pre-operatively, when assessed using a standardized scale, e.g. the Waterlow or Norton scales. Tissue viability may be impaired due to ischaemia, reduced nutritional intake because of anxiety and pain, resulting in weight loss, and, as already discussed, sensation and motor control may be reduced.

Patients' understanding

The Patients' Charter requires informed consent, and it is therefore necessary to assess patients' knowledge base in relation to their situation.

Nursing today aims to prevent disease and develop lifestyles that are healthy. Through education patients are empowered to be come actively involved in their own care and to take steps to reduce risk factors.

EXAMINATION

Basic examination equipment

The equipment used in assessment will include: a height-adjustable tilt couch or bed; documentation charts; a stethoscope; sphygmomanometer; oximeter urinalysis equipment; blood sugar monitor; chair weight scales; height measuring pole; tape measure for ankle circumference and a neurological tray containing equipment to assess sensitivity to hot and cold, pain and touch, motor reflex reaction and pupil reactions.

General examination

General examination may include the following:

- Recordable vital signs. Blood pressure should be taken in both arms, as calcification, stricture or occlusion of vessels or subclavian stenosis may in rare

---

When assessing acute peripheral arterial occlusion, the '6 Ps' will provide appropriate information:

- pain: position type, duration
- pallor: compare difference of colour in limbs
- pulse: audibility, quality, regularity, strength, absence
- paraesthesia: altered sensation, reduced/lost sensation
- paralysis: presence of paralysis
- poikilothermy: variation in body temperature, unrelated to environment.

cases give a variable result. Peripheral pulses and respiration—rate, rhythm and quality—must be checked.

• Auscultation for carotid or femoral bruits, cardiac murmurs and arrhythmias.

• Inspection of limbs and digits for changes suggestive of arterial disease—e.g. changes in colour such as cyanosis, dependent rubor (the phrase 'sunset leg' defines one which is red when dependent, but becomes pale on elevation), pallor and skin changes (for example, shiny hairless skin and microembolic phenomena presenting as patchy blue/cyanosed areas of skin, usually on the soles of the feet). Venous disease may be indicated by the presence of lipodermatosclerosis, ankle flare and atrophie blanche. The presence and site of ulceration, necrosis or gangrene will help to determine a differential diagnosis.

• Indications which suggest vasospasm, Raynaud's syndrome or phenomenon and previous frostbite—e.g. intermittent white fingers, coldness, numbness and pain in digits.

• Abdominal palpation for aortic aneurysm.

• Assessment of mobility (restricted by pain or arthritis).

• Assessment of nutritional status and special dietary needs.

Simple bedside investigations

• *Neurological assessment.* When patients present with arterial disease they may well give a history of transient ischaemic attacks or cerebrovascular accident resulting in neurological defects. The integrity of the reflex arcs may be tested using a patella hammer.

Fundoscopy will highlight any retinal changes, which are common in diabetic and hypertensive patients. However, areas of pallor in the discs, particularly if associated with visual field defects, indicate that thrombotic episodes may have arisen in the retinal artery. *Hollenhorst plaques*, seen on the retina, are bright reflective spots of cholesterol emboli from ulcerated plaques in the carotid artery, aortic arch or innominate artery. They may result in transient monocular blindness. Abnormalities of the visual fields should be noted pre-operatively to distinguish them from peri-operative events.

Although neurological examination will be undertaken by the medical staff prior to carotid surgery, it is important that the nurse be aware of any difficulties in swallowing, speech, power or sensation as a baseline pre-operatively and observe any postoperative changes. During carotid endarterectomy the surgical approach passes very near to some cranial nerves and damage to them may cause, for example, paralysis of the tongue (the hypoglossal nerve) or vocal cords (recurrent laryngeal nerve). For other nerves involved, see Chapter 12.

The 5% risk of stroke during this procedure should not be forgotten; postoperative neurological assessment will detect this.

Ischaemia can also have a damaging effect on the neurological system, resulting in a reduction or loss of sensation—especially in the feet—reduced motor control leading to a change in gait and loss of autonomic neurological activity. This leads to a reduction in sweating, which makes the feet dry and cracked. Simple tests will establish the status of local sensitivity. These may include:
— vibration using a tuning fork
— pin test for pain
— cotton wool for sensation
— hot and cold test-tubes for temperature.

• *Allen's test to indicate perfusion to the hand via the ulnar and radial arteries.* After the patient has been asked to make a fist, fingertip pressure is applied by the examiner to the ulnar and radial arteries. Observation of reperfusion to the hand is made as each artery is released separately. As most people are ulnar dominant, the radial artery is released first. This test will help to establish whether any ischaemic episode in the digits is due to pressure—as may be experienced in carpal tunnel syndrome—vasospastic disorders or occlusion of the major arteries of the arm.

- *Buerger's (pole) test to assess perfusion to the lower limbs.* Pulses are not normally lost on elevation in a limb free from disease, but they may be in a diseased limb. Where patients present with dependent rubor, calcification of arteries or oedema that prevents occlusion of the pulse in the lower limbs using a sphygmomanometer, the systolic pressure may be measured by elevating the leg during Doppler ultrasound or palpation of the pedal pulses and measuring the vertical height at which the pulse disappears. This height is proportional to the systolic pressure in the limb when it is horizontal. The vertical pole used for the purpose is calibrated in mmHg (Smith et al 1994).

- *Gentle pressure* applied to tissues or nail bed, to stimulate blanching. When this is released the duration of time taken to refill the capillary beds can be observed. Normal recovery time is 3 seconds.

- *Doppler assessment* to ascertain the presence of pedal pulses and ankle brachial pressure index, as discussed below.

- *Trendelenburg's test for evaluation of varicosities below the knee.* With the patient supine, the leg is elevated, thus emptying the veins, and a soft rubber cuff is applied below the knee. When the patient stands up, the varicosities are observed. If they refill immediately, this indicates that the valves in the perforators are incompetent. However, if the varicosities only refill when the cuff is released, the indication is that only the valves of the saphenous vein are incompetent.

- *Perthes' test to check the patency and competence of the perforators.* A cuff is applied below the knee while the patient is standing. The varicosities will be evident. The patient is then asked to plantarflex the foot repeatedly; this, by working the calf muscle pump, should empty the peripheral veins. Failure to do so demonstrates that the perforators are incompetent or blocked.

- *Homans' sign* for the presence of deep venous thrombosis. This procedure is designed to put deep veins in the calf on the stretch. The patient lies supine with straight legs and the foot is forcibly dorsiflexed. If this produces pain in the calf, the test is positive.

- *Ward urinalysis.* This should be mandatory, particularly to check for glucose, ketones and proteins.

- *Ward blood glucose test* to indicate hyper- or hypoglycaemia.

- *Weight and height measurement.* Baseline readings will provide useful information, e.g. to calculate body mass index and the possible need for weight modification, monitoring oedema or in assessment for wheelchairs.

- *Classical signs for dehydration.* These should be identified early by, for example, monitoring the specific gravity of the urine, measuring fluid balance and observing the clinical status of the skin and serial levels of blood urea.

> Hand-held Doppler ultrasound is a useful tool:
> - demonstrates arterial blood flow
> - defines arterial pressure
> - denotes venous reflux.

> Bedside assessment of blood flow
>
> Arterial
> - Allen's test
> - Buerger pole test
> - hand-held doppler/ABPI
> - reperfusion time
>
> Venous
> - Trendelenburg's test
> - Perthes' test
> - Homans' sign
> - Doppler reflux.

OVERVIEW OF THE VASCULAR LABORATORY

Any major centre dealing with vascular surgery needs access to a vascular laboratory's equipment and resources. In the vascular field, radiology and surgery work closely together in both diagnosis and treatment.

The laboratory will include facilities for blood and urine screening.

Blood screening

A *full blood count* will yield information on a number of scores. Without a normal *haemoglobin* level (at least below 100 g/l) there is inadequate oxygen-carrying capacity to withstand a prolonged anaesthetic; low haemoglobin will, moreover, impede wound healing and may contribute to leg ulceration. It could also warn of coexisting disease, for example, malignancy. A haemoglobin level greater than 180 g/l indicates polycythaemia, with an increase in viscosity.

The *mean corpuscular volume (MCV)* is the measurement of the size of the red blood cells. The MCV value in the presence of low haemoglobin will help identify the type of anaemia involved. Small cells (microcytosis) indicate iron deficiency, perhaps due to chronic blood loss or poor nutrition. Normal sized cells (normocytosis) in anaemia indicate a chronic disease such as rheumatoid arthritis or renal failure. Abnormally large cells (macrocytosis) suggest folate or vitamin B_{12} deficiency (as in pernicious anaemia), though they can also be a sign of chronic alcoholism.

Measurement of *mean corpuscular haemoglobin (MCH)* together with the MCV will enable one to calculate the *mean corpuscular haemoglobin concentration (MCHC)* which helps to distinguish between abnormally sized cells and cells which lack haemoglobin. Lastly, the full blood count includes the *number* of red cells.

A raised *white cell count* is usually indicative of the presence of infection.

Assessment of platelets and a coagulation screen are necessary routine procedures before major surgery. Monitoring these indices in patients who have been anticoagulated or who have coexisting liver disease is particularly important.

The *erythrocyte sedimentation rate (ESR)* by itself does not provide a diagnosis. However, where this is raised it usually indicates the presence of inflammation, but may also suggest collagen disease, malignancy or anaemia.

Antibody screening is important for differential diagnosis in patients with leg ulcers and suspected vasculitic ulceration—e.g. patients with a history of rheumatoid arthritis.

A *biochemical profile* will highlight renal abnormalities (urea, creatinine) and electrolyte disturbances which may predispose to cardiac arrhythmias, hypertension, headaches, confusion or reduced bowel motility.

A reduced *serum albumin* will delay the process of wound healing. The reduction may be due to a heavy wound exudate loss, as seen in patients with leg ulceration, or to poor nutritional intake.

Raised *cholesterol* (and triglycerides) may have been identified, as hypercholesterolaemia is associated with atherosclerosis. Provided this has been recorded there is no need to repeat the test, as the level does not rise significantly after the age of 25.

Blood screening for smoking markers will enable the clinician to assess the cooperation of the patient in stopping smoking, which will enhance his or her postoperative chances.

Arterial blood gases allow assessment of PO_2, PCO_2 and pH levels. The ratio of bicarbonate to carbonic acid will determine the presence of acidosis or alkalosis. A pH of less than 7.35 indicates that the patient is acidotic and a pH of greater than 7.45 indicates that he or she is alkalotic. 3–5 $kPaCO_2$ and 11–15 $kPaO_2$ is normal. Should the PO_2 fall below 11 kPa, hypoxia is present. Breathlessness occurs when there are abnormalities of acid-base balance. Postoperatively, the analysis of blood gases may also be required to ascertain the cause of such breathlessness.

Any history of chest pain, previous cardiac surgery or shortness of breath in the pre-operative period warrants the measurement of *cardiac enzymes*, especially where a patient is known to have ischaemic heart disease. Sixty-three per cent of vascular surgical patients in a recent study showed evidence of coronary artery disease (Taylor 1992). In patients who have undergone aortic aneurysm repair, myocardial infarction is not uncommon around the third day after the operation, and routine screening may be helpful in ensuring early recognition and treatment. It needs to be borne in mind that the creatine phosphokinase (CPK) may be raised

Useful blood screening tests:

- haematology
  — FBC: Hb, MCV, MCH, MCHC, number of RBCs
  — ESR
  — clotting screen
  — antibody screen
  — B_{12} folate, ferritin
- biochemistry
  — U/Es
  — creatinine
  — calcium
  — total protein: albumin + globulin
- cardiac enzymes
- lipids
- thyroid studies
- liver function tests
- glucose and HbA_1C.

anyway, owing to the surgical muscular trauma, so one needs to measure the more specific enzyme levels for cardiac muscle damage, such as lactate dehydrogenase (LDH) and the cardiospecific enzyme creatine kinase myocardial band, which is only identified when trauma is specific to the cardiac muscle.

Prior to vascular surgery blood will be *grouped and cross-matched*. The figures below are only a guide to the number of units to be saved, which may vary, depending on the severity of the patient's condition and consultant preference:

- carotid endarterectomy: 2 units
- reconstructive surgery involving the aorta: 6 units
- other reconstructive surgery: 4 units
- aortic aneurysm repair: 6–8 units.

Dehydration should be identified early by its classical signs—for example, dryness and flaccidity of the skin. The specific gravity of urine may be elevated and fluid output may be significantly less than fluid intake. Serial levels of blood urea may also be raised.

SPECIFIC INVESTIGATIONS

Pulmonary

A standard pre-operative chest X-ray to identify potential respiratory or cardiac problems is usually performed.

Peak flow/vitalography will enable assessment of pulmonary function. Measurements may be taken and compared with standard values for height and age of *vital capacity* (the amount of air exhaled from full inspiration to full expiration), *tidal volume* (the amount of air exhaled in relaxed breathing) and *functional residual capacity* (the difference between vital capacity and tidal volume). If these are significantly abnormal, or if the *forced expiratory volume in 1 second (FEV$_1$)* is less than 30% of normal values, or if carbon dioxide tension in the arterial blood is greater than 5.5 kPa, then there is a significant risk of post-operative pulmonary complications. In these cases the response to bronchodilators would be helpful additional information.

Serial oximetry or occasionally measurement of other blood gases peri- and post-operatively will allow objective assessment of the need for oxygen therapy or assisted ventilation.

> There is a potentially increased postoperative pulmonary risk associated with:
>
> - FEV$_1$ < 30%
> - arterial tissue tension > 5.5 kPa
> - significant difference between tidal volume and functional residual capacity.

Renal

Renal disease may be suspected if there is a urine output of less than 30 ml per hour or if it is suggested by the past medical history, or biochemistry results as above. The presence of protein, leucocytes or nitrites suggests infection. Blood may be indicative of glomerular renal dysfunction. Metabolic or diabetic ketoacidosis may be indicated in the presence of a positive ward urinalysis for glucose and ketones. Dipstick urinalysis should be mandatory on a first assessment for any vascular patient to establish the presence of glucose, ketones, protein or raised specific gravity.

> Urinalysis should be mandatory on any first assessment. Normal output per hour is expected to be around 30 ml.

Cardiovascular assessment

Prior to any cardio/peripherovascular investigation any history of coronary heart disease or breathlessness must be recognized, and blood pressure, pulse rate and rhythm should be assessed. Strict protocols need to be observed during any procedures that will put the heart under stress, e.g. treadmill exercise tolerance. If abnormal changes are noted in respiration, blood pressure or pulse rate and rhythm, the test should be aborted immediately.

Electrocardiogram

As with all major operations, a pre-operative *electrocardiogram* is essential.

Prior to major vascular surgery, the heart needs to be placed under stress to assess its ability to cope with the increased strain placed upon it peri-operatively. This may be performed using one or more of the following investigations.

A *treadmill echogram* non-invasively assesses left ventricular size and function by measuring movement of the ventricular walls and valves in a two-dimensional mode, or *treadmill electrocardiography*, running an ECG continuously during tread-mill movement. Alternatively, in patients with claudication, pharmacological stressor such as dobutamine may be used instead of exercise.

Radioactive thallium imaging uses the drug *dipyridamole* (whose effects can be reversed by aminophylline) to stress the heart pharmacologically. Intravenous thallium—administered after the dipyridamole, and prior to scanning—is taken up by the myocardium; a lack of up-take may illustrate ischaemia at rest. After two to three hours' rest, imaging is repeated and comparisons are drawn between the two studies. There is usually sufficient thallium in the system to enable the repeat scan to be informative. Any arrhythmias are noted.

Where this test is positive there is a 30% predicted risk of a coronary ischaemic event after the operation and it is wise to investigate further using *coronary angiography* (Hallett 1995). This is only used in selected cases as it may induce myocardial infarction.

Central venous pressure may be recorded in order to ascertain the fluid load on the heart.

In order to obtain the pressure in the right atrium a catheter is inserted through a peripheral vein to the vena cava. Pressure in the left atrium is measured by inserting a *Swan–Ganz catheter*. This may also be inserted through a peripheral vein and then taken through the right heart until it lodges in a small vessel in the lung. The pressure at this point is the same as the pressure in the pulmonary vein or left atrium.

A manometer, with a normal range of between 2 and 7 cm of saline, is used to measure the central venous pressure. Should the reading rise above this normal range, it is indicative of fluid overload and right heart failure.

> Assessment of cardiac function
>
> - electrocardiogram
> - treadmill electrocardiogram
> - treadmill echogram
> - radioactive thallium imaging.

Non-invasive peripheral vascular studies

Doppler ultrasound

The Austrian Christian Doppler (1803–1853) was the first to describe how the pitch of a sound rises as its source nears the observer, and then falls as it moves away from the observer—as, for example, in the sound of a train moving towards a station and then passing through. This change in frequency is called the 'Doppler shift'. The Doppler signal has been used in various medical applications since the 1960s. Doppler signal analysis is a useful and easy guide which can be used as an adjunctive diagnostic tool in both arterial and venous disease. It should only be used in conjunction with a full medical and nursing history and examination. More sophisticated investigations may be required to confirm the diagnosis.

Ultrasonic high-frequency sounds are emitted from a piezoelectric crystal transducer which is contained in a hand-held probe. This vibrates when charged with an electric current, emitting a high-pitched sound wave which bounces off the erythrocytes in the flowing blood; because of the 'Doppler effect' the returning echo is at a slightly lower frequency. Another crystal in the probe picks up this echo wave as it moves towards the probe and compares it with the emitted wave, translating the difference into an audible sound. The frequency of that sound therefore varies according to the characteristics of the flow velocity. The differential between the emitted signal and that heard represents the Doppler shift.

Doppler probes are available in different frequencies. The lower the frequency the deeper the waves will penetrate. Therefore, a 4 or 5 mHz probe is better for assessing deep veins or arteries and an 8 mHz probe is more suitable for peripheral vessels.

Doppler ultrasound is indicated for identifying the level of occlusion and the presence of distal pulses before and after aortic aneurysm and bypass reconstructive surgery, and for aiding diagnosis in patients with varicose veins and leg/foot ulceration. The possibility of ischaemia must be eliminated before leg ulcers are treated using compression. More detailed analysis of the significance of ankle brachial pressure index (ABPI) values in relation to the management of patients with leg ulcers may be found in Chapter 6.

The foot pulses that can be located in the healthy person are those corresponding to the posterior tibial, anterior tibial, peroneal and dorsalis pedis arteries (Ch. 1). Barnhorst and Barner (1968) found the dorsalis pedis pulse to be congenitally absent in up to 12% of normal people. However, a study performed by Brearley et al (1992) demonstrated that it is only genuinely absent in up to 1.9% of normal subjects, and that the failure to detect a posterior tibial signal is rare.

Procedure for Doppler assessment It is becoming standard practice for appropriately trained nurses to undertake Doppler arterial perfusion assessment, measuring the resting ankle brachial pressure index as an indicator of the degree of arterial perfusion. A hand-held Doppler can be used merely to ascertain the presence of pedal pulses, for example following reconstructive bypass surgery, or to assess the degree of arterial pressure in the distal vessels (Fig. 5.1).

Measuring a resting ankle brachial pressure index (ABPI) This procedure will establish the ratio between arterial pressure at the ankle and that in the brachial artery. A simple hand-held Doppler ultrasound probe is used in place of a stethoscope to monitor the systolic pressures. A normal resting pressure index is considered to range from 0.9 to 1.2, i.e. 90–120% perfusion.

The procedure should be explained to the patient and whenever possible he or she should be supine during assessment of the ABPI so that the brachial and ankle pulses lie in the same plane. If this is not possible owing to dyspnoea or arthritis, the patient should be made as comfortable as possible in the semirecumbent position. The position of the patient during assessment should be recorded, as the fact that the patient is sitting up or that the legs are dependent can affect the supply of blood to the distal vessels.

The ABPI is a *resting* pressure index, and therefore allowing the patient to relax for 15 minutes before the recording will allow more accurate assessment.

With the aid of the Doppler probe, the systolic brachial pressure is monitored in both arms on a first assessment. This is important, as arterial disease is not specific and may present in either of the brachial arteries, giving variable readings in each arm. The sphygmomanometer cuff should be long enough to ensure that 80% of the circumference of the upper arm or ankle can be covered by the bladder of the cuff.

Again, with the use of the Doppler probe, posterior tibial, anterior tibial and peroneal pulses are identified where audible and their individual pressures recorded. It is important to ensure that the cuff of the sphygmomanometer is placed around the ankle. Even when patients present with leg ulcers around the ankle, Doppler assessment can be undertaken by first covering the ulcer with a sterile protective lining: for example, the disposable dressing bag can be used, once the bottom has been cut off, to make a tube through which the leg can be placed, or a dressing towel can be placed over the wound. This will help to prevent cross-infection and soiling of the sphygmomanometer cuff. Should the ulcer lie in the immediate area

The resting ankle brachial pressure index is a comparison of the blood pressure in the arm with that in the leg:

- A normal index is 0.9–1.2
- A pressure index of < 0.8 denotes ischaemia
- A pressure index of > 1.3 may indicate false readings due to calcification or inflammation in the arteries.

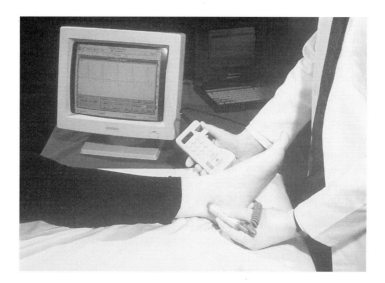

Fig. 5.1 Using a hand-held Doppler probe. (Reproduced with kind permission from Huntleigh Nesbit Evans Healthcare.)

of the pedal pulses, it can be protected with a water-based dressing such as *gelperm wet*, which is 90% water and therefore permeable to the ultrasound wave.

Doppler values In the healthy individual with no arterial disease, the systolic pressure in the brachial artery should be equal to that in the ankle. The pressure in the ankle is divided by the pressure in the arm to ascertain the resting ankle brachial pressure index (ABPI):

$$\frac{\text{ankle pressure}}{\text{brachial pressure}}$$

It follows that normal ABPI is 1.0, i.e. 100% blood flow. Any recording less than 0.8 (80%) indicates the presence of ischaemia. A ratio greater than 1.3 may be indicative of calcification or oedema which has given rise to falsely elevated readings. Elevation of the leg will show whether there is sufficient arterial pressure to maintain a pulsatile signal on elevation and therefore whether or not the recorded ABPI is a true reading.

Currently there is much debate as to whether the highest or the lowest pressure in the limbs should be used to calculate ABPI. The literature advocates using the highest arm and highest pedal pressure. However, it may be more prudent to take full account of the presenting history and, if there is any indication of arterial or small vessel disease, to err on the side of caution and take the pressures which allow for the largest safety margin. Any concern regarding accurate ABPI should lead the nurse to ensure that the patient has a vascular referral and full assessment before using compression.

Where calcification of vessels or oedema exists, the pressure ratio may be elevated, as described above. Microvascular disease may coexist with what appears to be a normal ABPI, and therefore it is essential always to take a full history. This will eliminate the possibility of inflammation of the small vessels, as in vasculitic disorders, such as rheumatoid arthritis, or calcification of such vessels, as in diabetes, before compression therapy is applied to patients presenting with leg ulcers or varicose eczema.

In young, healthy people, the arteries in the leg are elastic and supply a predominantly muscular tissue bed, which naturally offers some resistance to blood flow. There are three specific phases to each pulse. In systole, whilst the heart contracts pressure is exerted on the flow, and the blood accelerates along the artery in a forward direction away from the heart, causing the vessel to expand. Then, during diastole there is relaxation of the vessels, and flow. Finally, the blood continues to move forward again. This pattern is demonstrable in the normal three-part flow wave, as seen in Figure 5.2. Thus the Doppler signal is described as a *triphasic sound*. Peripheral vascular disease changes the normal triphasic wave form. In the presence of mild to moderate disease it becomes *biphasic* because the artery is less elastic, and therefore a more muffled sound with two components is emitted, as the resting part of the diastolic signal is lost. In the presence of severe disease the signal becomes *monophasic*, sounding more like a pulsatile wind rushing through the vessels. The systolic wave becomes more flattened on a printout, as there is less pressure on the vessel wall owing to the reduced perfusion through the occluded vessel. As the major vessels become totally occluded so the signal will fade away, as there is no blood velocity for the ultrasound to bounce off.

The audible signal heard in bidirectional flow can be enhanced by the use of stereophonic headphones, which transmit each phase of the signal to alternate ears.

Hand-held Doppler ultrasound may be equipped with a software package to enable complete vascular studies to be documented and saved in a patient database or as hard copy printouts (Fig. 5.2).

Recording *segmental pressures* along the leg may help to define the position of occlusion. A pressure difference of 30 mmHg between each segment represents a significant stenosis in that region.

A treadmill is a useful adjunct to hand-held Doppler ultrasound studies in assessing exercise tolerance in claudicant patients. After the ABPI has initially been

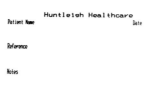

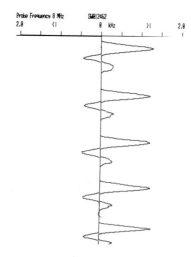

Fig. 5.2 Doppler printout wave forms. (Reproduced with kind permission from Huntleigh Nesbit Evans Healthcare.)

recorded, the patient is asked to walk on a treadmill which runs at a speed of approximately 2–3 k/h with an incline of 10°. The test will demonstrate the distance a patient is able to walk before experiencing claudication, i.e. pain in the feet, legs or buttocks induced by lack of oxygen perfusion to tissues in the presence of arterial disease (Fig. 5.3). The distance and time taken before the first onset of pain (claudication) is noted.

The patient continues with the test until unable to tolerate the claudication pain. At this stage, he or she is laid supine or semirecumbent and the ABPI is reassessed. The length of recovery time to pre-treadmill pressure assessment is noted, along with any differential in pre- and post-exercise ABPI. In the presence of significant arterial disease, pulses may disappear totally.

> Claudication may be assessed using a treadmill and Doppler ultrasound. The speed, distance and time walked is measured. A drop in ABPI post-treadmill assessment is indicative of occlusion. Regular follow-up monitoring can give an indication of the progress of arterial disease.

Duplex scanning

Sonic ultrasound flow detection is used in the assessment of arterial and venous flow ranges from simple *'brightness mode'* (B-mode) to more complex *colour flow duplex ultrasonic scanners*.

B-mode Two-dimensional images of tissues are produced on a screen (Fig. 5.4). The denser the tissue, the deeper the shade of grey presented. Position and length of stenosis can be detected non-invasively, but not enough information is given regarding retrograde flow, as B-mode cannot give any indication of direction of flow.

Colour flow arterial duplex This provides a visual illustration of 'Doppler shift'. It is more useful than B-mode ultrasound scanning in the assessment of arterial occlusion and venous insufficiency as it clearly demonstrates flow direction. The presence of moving venous or arterial blood and the velocity of blood

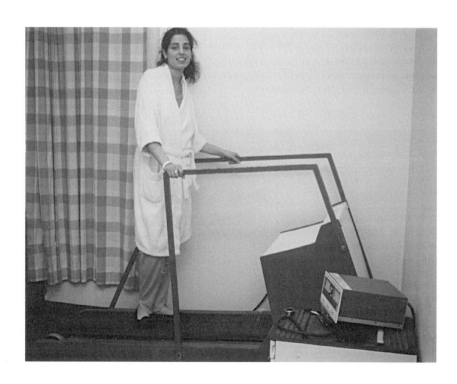

Fig. 5.3 Patient undergoing Doppler treadmill assessment.

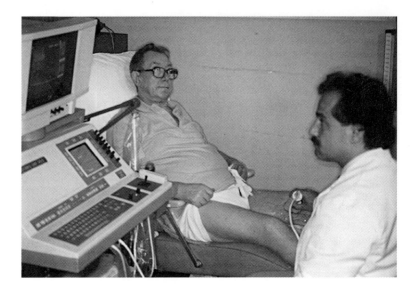

Fig. 5.4 B-mode duplex scanner. (Reproduced with kind permission from Mr Paterson, Good Hope NHS Trust.)

In colour duplex images:

- red indicates flow of blood towards the probe
- blue indicates flow of blood away from the probe, resulting from occlusion.

flow indicates more clearly areas and lengths of stenosis and the presence of arteriovenous shunts (Fig. 5.5).

The direction of flow is picked up by the ultrasonic probe and displayed on a screen as red for blood flowing towards the probe and as blue for blood flowing away from it. Normal arterial flow speed is 40–45 cm/s. Where there is a stenosis the velocity of the flow increases and this is demonstrated by a change in colour from red to orange and then to yellow, or from blue to aqua to white. Post-stenotic turbulence is depicted as a mixture of all the colours. Doppler *spectrum sound* produces a higher-frequency sound where vessels bifurcate and over areas of stenosis where the velocity of flow increases.

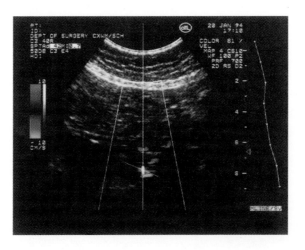

Fig. 5.5 Printout from a colour duplex scanner showing arterial flow through a vessel.

In the presence of an arteriovenous fistula red and blue may be seen together.

Portable ultrasound

This facilitates screening for aortic aneurysms, as a service can be offered to local health centres for males over the age of 65. Currently there is an authoritative multicentre study under way in Chichester aimed at assessing value of screening in reducing the mortality rates in the 7–8% of men who present with aortic aneurysm. Studies on the cost-effectiveness of screening are of value in determining whether or not this is a worthwhile venture.

The indications for conventional surgical intervention in cases of aortic aneurysm are (a) if there has been an increase in the aortic diameter of more than 1 cm in 1 year, or (b) if the diameter is greater than 5 cm. The general health of the patient is also taken into consideration. Currently these margins are under review. Should a patient be found to have a terminal illness, the offer of surgery may be withdrawn.

Carotid ultrasonic scanning can highlight the potential risk of stroke in cases where carotid arteries are found to be stenosed. More than 70% stenosis may be regarded as an indication for carotid endarterectomy.

> Duplex demonstrates colour shifts with increasing velocity through a partial stenosis. Where the stenosis is complete, as in a DVT, colour disappears.

> Portable ultrasound scanning for AAA and carotid stenosis will permit early detection of the potential need for surgery in a bid to reduce the incidence of AAA rupture and stroke.

Transcranial Doppler (TCD)

This is a useful means of determining the status of the intracranial circulation. Although in its infancy, TCD may be used to assess the patency of individual intracranial arteries and the presence of collaterals or occlusions.

Computed tomography (CT)

CT is an accessible way of assessing vascular patients at risk of aortic and peripheral aneurysms or those presenting with complications following the insertion of grafts in reconstruction bypass surgery.

There are no complications with this non-invasive technique. CT scans make measurements which are perpendicular to the body. Aneurysms are often tortuous, so when they are measured at an oblique angle an overestimation of their size may be obtained.

3D multiseeded CT angiography

This may be found in some of the larger vascular centres where a spiral scanner is available. It allows a clear depiction of the volume of the individual structures to be identified, giving an indication of the size of the aneurysm and its position in relation to other structures.

Magnetic resonance imaging (MRI)

This has the benefit of providing clear pictures when patients are being screened for an aortic aneurysm or graft complications. Prior to the 1960s, arteriography was the only means of assessing vascular problems in depth. However, with the advent of ultrasound, CT and MRI, arteriography now tends to be reserved for the assessment of peripheral vascular disease and radiographic therapy.

Positron emission tomography (PET)

Whereas MRI examinations efficiently pick out the shapes of structures, so PET distinguishes substances. It will therefore produce an image which can be programmed to show healthy against ischaemic tissue, differences in oxygen saturation or a vast array of metabolic changes. The technique is to inject biologically active substances labelled with radioactive isotopes which emit particles called

MRI scans distinguish shapes
PET scans distinguish substances.

positrons, to allow these to permeate the tissues and then to map out the distribution. The use of PET in vascular surgery is associated with tissue viability.

Invasive arterial studies

Angiography

Although an invasive technique that carries risks, angiography, also known as arteriography, still remains the investigation of choice for exploring the status of the main arteries. It gives a clear and definitive diagnosis when there is a need to distinguish between occlusive and vasospastic disorders. It demonstrates the presence of collateral blood vessels and the feasibility of surgery. Arteriography is also used to allow therapeutic intervention if thrombolysis or angioplasty are warranted (Fig. 5.6).

Preparation for angiography

- Informed consent needs to be gained.
- Prior to any invasive radiological investigation requiring the use of a radiographic contrast medium, previous known allergies should be ascertained and the radiologist informed.
- In some centres the puncture site will be shaved prior to the procedure.
- The patient should be nil by mouth for 6 hours prior to the procedure. This precaution should be taken in case embolectomy is required as a result of the dislodgement of plaque during the procedure.

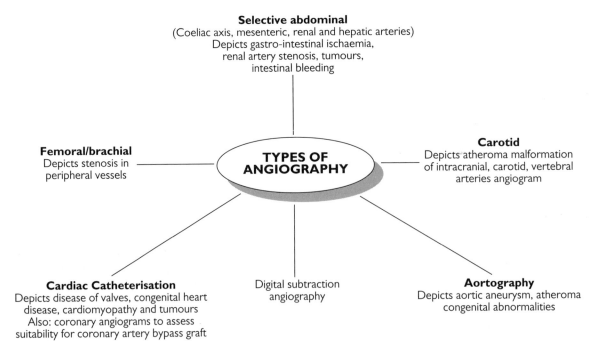

Selective abdominal
(Coeliac axis, mesenteric, renal and hepatic arteries)
Depicts gastro-intestinal ischaemia,
renal artery stenosis, tumours,
intestinal bleeding

Femoral/brachial
Depicts stenosis in
peripheral vessels

TYPES OF ANGIOGRAPHY

Carotid
Depicts atheroma malformation
of intracranial, carotid, vertebral
arteries angiogram

Cardiac Catheterisation
Depicts disease of valves, congenital heart
disease, cardiomyopathy and tumours
Also: coronary angiograms to assess
suitability for coronary artery bypass graft

Digital subtraction
angiography

Aortography
Depicts aortic aneurysm, atheroma
congenital abnormalities

Fig. 5.6 Types of angiography.

- Baseline observations of vital signs should be recorded.
- A theatre gown is normally worn to protect the patient's clothing.
- It is important to ensure all notes and prescription charts are taken with the patient to the X-ray department.

In 1953, Seldinger introduced the technique of inserting a needle into the vessel to allow access to a guidewire through the lumen of the vessel. Repeated changes of catheters can then be safely fed into the vessel over the guidewire, which is then withdrawn after each catheter insertion. Radiographic contrast medium is perfused into the vessel under pressure. This should be non-ionic, which is less painful than an ionic medium. Careful observation of the patient is maintained during this procedure. The femoral arteries are usually the vessels of choice as they offer the safest access, unless this route is contraindicated owing to complete stenosis or previous surgery. It is not uncommon for a femoral artery to be approached from the contralateral side so reducing the risk of puncturing a vessel that will later be involved in bypass surgery. Also, if there is an occlusion which would respond to angioplasty or thrombolysis it is easier to cross over the aorto-iliac bifurcation and direct the catheter distally.

Patients should be warned that they will experience a warm sensation throughout their body and that they may feel as though they are micturating. These are normal body responses to the contrast medium. A video picture will allow immediate access to information and this can be kept as a hard-copy arteriogram. Such pictures are invaluable during vascular surgery as a means of recognizing the geography of the vessels and their condition.

Following the procedure, pressure is applied to the puncture site for at least 10 to 20 minutes using a piece of sterile gauze held in place by a firm hand. The patient should not be left alone. Blood pressure and pulse are monitored frequently and the patient is asked to lie still for at least 6 hours to reduce the risk of post-procedure haemorrhage. He or she should be encouraged to drink in order to flush out contrast medium from the kidneys.

Digital subtraction angiography (DSA) The principle of digital subtraction is that greater clarity of image can be achieved. If a straight X-ray (which is a 'negative' photograph) is held up to the light superimposed on its 'positive' equivalent, light and dark will cancel each other out. If only one of the two films includes the contrast passing through the arteries, then the picture of the artery is the only feature demonstrated (Fig. 5.7).

Access may be gained through a peripheral vein, with the tip of the catheter placed in the right atrium. Contrast is released and flows through the pulmonary circulation, back through the left heart, into the aorta and on to the arterial system, where any stenosis is identified.

Although digital subtraction was initially designed to enable contrast to be infused via a peripheral vein, many centres find the contrast too dilute to give the clarity of picture they are seeking. Therefore, arterial access is used unless arteries are severely occluded and access is not possible.

Risks associated with arteriography These include nausea, haematoma, haemorrhage, pseudoaneurysm, anaphylaxis, sensitivity reaction, radiographic contrast-induced allergy, the dislodgement of thrombus, blood/air embolus formation and initiation of arrhythmias. The patient needs to be made aware that this is an invasive procedure and that there are associated risks, although these are as low as 1%, with a 0.5% risk of mortality.

Risks of arteriography:

- haematoma
- pseudoaneurysm
- anaphylaxis and sensitivity reaction
- arrhythmias.

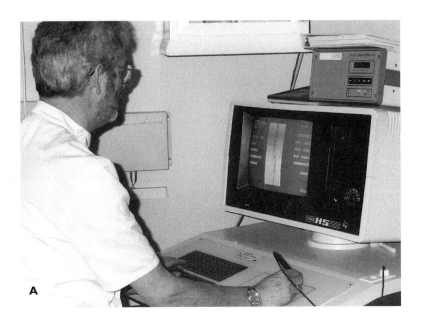

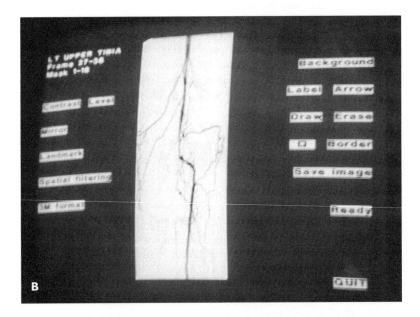

Fig. 5.7 Digital subtraction angiography is undertaken to highlight relevant structures, allowing a clearer picture to be obtained. (**A**) Screen and operator. (**B**) Close-up of screen.

VENOUS STUDIES

Doppler ultrasound

In some centres hand-held Doppler assessment is used in patients with varicose veins to determine venous reflux in the presence of valvular incompetence. This is a simple bedside test which can be performed while the patient is standing. Once the vein has been located with the Doppler probe, pressure is applied to the leg and a whooshing noise is heard as the leg is squeezed and venous blood ejected from the vessel. In the absence of venous incompetence there will be no venous reflux signal on release of pressure, as the valves prevent this.

Venous duplex

Duplex is an accurate means of detecting a deep vein thrombosis, and has replaced venography in centres which have a duplex scanner. The sonographer looks for lack of movement in the vein (a black area), the presence of material in the lumen, lack of compressibility in the vein and a lack of the swelling effect that Valsalva's manoeuvre normally creates.

Figure 5.8 demonstrates venous incompetence at the saphenofemoral vein. The patient was examined whilst standing. As the calf is squeezed, venous blood flows towards the heart (illustrated by the first wave form below the line). On release of the calf there is significant venous reflux, lasting for 1.5 seconds (illustrated by the second wave form above the line).

Venogram

This is indicated when venous duplexing is unable to provide a definitive diagnosis of deep vein thrombosis. Prior to venous bypass or venous valve reconstruction surgery, venogram will be the investigation of choice, as greater clarity will be gained.

There is a 3% risk of allergic reactions associated with venographic studies, e.g. thrombophlebitis which may be contrast-induced or due to extravasation at the puncture site. This could lead to a deep vein thrombosis. There is less than a 1% chance of major reactions such as hypotension or bronchospasm.

During the procedure the patient is placed at a 45° tilt with the head up and non-weight-bearing, as weight-bearing would reduce the efficiency of venous filling, due to the contraction of the gastrocnemius and soleus muscles.

A 21-gauge needle is inserted into the vein—usually on the dorsum of the foot—through which contrast medium can be injected under pressure. Exposures of the vessels can then be made segmentally at the level of the ankle, calf and thigh. Following the procedure the leg is elevated to aid venous return.

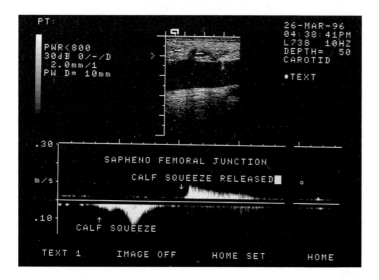

Fig. 5.8 Venous duplex showing saphenofemoral reflux.

Plethysmography

This is the measurement of changes in the volume of a limb, and can be used to determine venous flow. Plethysmography obtains information non-invasively by various means, including measuring the circumference of the calf with a strain gauge and measuring the electrical resistance across the limb with an impedance meter (blood is a good conductor of electricity). Alternatively, air plethysmography depends on monitors within an air-filled cuff applied to the lower limb.

Results are recorded before, during and after exercise. A normal result demonstrates a drop in pressure as the calf muscle empties during exercise and a gradual return to normal 30 to 40 seconds after movement has stopped. If the deep vein is occluded and the collaterals are insufficient to convey adequate venous return, the drop in pressure is much less and the return to normal levels is slower. In extreme cases the pressure actually increases temporarily.

Direct measurement of venous pressure

The pressure which the calf muscles exert on the distal veins may be measured directly by inserting a fine needle into a foot vein with a pressure-measuring device (oncometer). Results are interpreted in the same way as for plethsymography.

Repeat investigations

Some of the above investigations may be performed as an outpatient procedure and repeated on the day of admission. Where patients present with coexisting renal disease or are taking anticoagulation therapy, it is important to repeat blood screening on the day before surgery. Patients undergoing carotid endarterectomy may require a repeat carotid scan on the day of surgery; ECG, chest X-ray and echocardiograms may also be repeated prior to surgery, depending on the status of the patient and consultant preference.

Patients attending for vascular assessment need to be aware that the procedures are for the purposes of investigation and are not therapeutic.

THE IMPORTANCE OF ASSESSMENT FOR PATIENTS WITH LEG ULCERATION

Before the middle ages it was thought that ulcers encouraged the release of dangerous and foul humours (Underwood 1983). However, today we know this not to be so, and the anatomy, physiology and aetiology of ulceration needs to be recognized by the practitioner in order to ensure correct differential diagnosis and management, and thereby aid the process of healing.

Holistic assessment is critical to the prevention of further damage, to the maintenance of general health and to the success of healing. It should ensure that care is sensitive, responsive, relevant and safe, meeting individual needs cost-effectively within given resources.

Cameron (1991) recognizes that the consequence of incorrect diagnosis of leg ulcers can be disastrous for patients. 'Accurate assessment will help to eliminate or reduce the perpetuating factors' (Ertl 1993), as well as to ensure appropriate planning for the treatment of the ulcer, with modifications being made as needed on the basis of regular evaluation.

The nurse's responsibility for the assessment of patients with leg ulcers

Cullum and Roe (1995) state that 98% of district nurses have responsibility for leg ulcer patients. Many decisions in treatment are delegated to the nurse as an autonomous practitioner (McIntosh 1979).

An alarming fact revealed by Cullum is that nurses often take responsibility for diagnosis, as demonstrated by an unpublished audit carried out in Stockport; this showed that 52% of cases were diagnosed by the nurse as against 25% by the GP or consultant. Sadly, this study found that 51% of the diagnoses had been made on the appearance of the ulcer alone (Cullum 1994). If nurses are managing wounds autonomously they need to ensure that their assessment is made from a comprehensive and sound knowledge base. Moffatt et al (1994) carried out a study in Bedfordshire which, disturbingly, shows that 38% of patients were left undiagnosed and the ulcer was classified as 'disease of unknown aetiology' because the nurse was unable to identify it.

If nurses cannot determine the aetiology of an ulcer owing to lack of knowledge, the Scope of Professional Practice makes provision for refusal to carry out a procedure. However, it goes on to state that this deficit has to be rectified, and in the meantime it is essential that the patient be referred to someone who has sufficient knowledge to carry out treatment. 'It is imperative that patients with leg ulcers be given the benefit of a medical diagnosis and an in-depth nursing assessment so that an appropriate and effective plan of management may be developed' (Roe et al 1993).

Where, in spite of accurate assessment and a sound knowledge base, nurses are unable to identify the aetiology, they are responsible for bringing this to the attention of clinicians and for ensuring that an accurate diagnosis is obtained, possibly by means of more sophisticated arterial and venous investigations, e.g. arteriography, venous duplex and blood screening.

However, tests which the nurse will be able to perform are screening for raised blood sugar, identifying wound infections (if suggested by the presence of pus, pyrexia or cellulitis) by sending swabs for culture and sensitivity, and using Doppler ultrasound to assess arterial sufficiency. While nurses do not claim to be clinicians, a sound knowledge base will protect the patient from the potential harm caused by inappropriate treatment planning, and may allow earlier identification of risk factors and disease entities.

Leg ulcer assessment

Factors to be considered during assessment of patients with leg ulcers are highlighted in Figure 5.9 and Table 5.1.

Table 5.1 What are we assessing?

Assessment	Rationale
Past medical history	An indicator of conditions associated with leg ulcer, e.g. diabetes, CHD, PE
Risk assessment	Identify potential hazards, e.g. smoking, obesity
Immediate cause of the ulcer	Identify minor trauma, foreign bodies, ill-fitting shoes
Differential diagnosis	Line of treatment will depend on accurate diagnosis. Important to ensure arterial ulcers are not treated with compression (Moffatt 1994)
Presentation of wound bed	Dressings/treatment will only be effective if used appropriately
General health status	Healing may be affected by general factors which need addressing, e.g. nutrition
Social circumstances	Poverty, poor housing, loneliness, low social class have all been demonstrated to delay wound healing and therefore need attention (Cullum 1994)
Day-to-day activities	Identify potential and actual problems, so enabling appropriate supports to be implemented

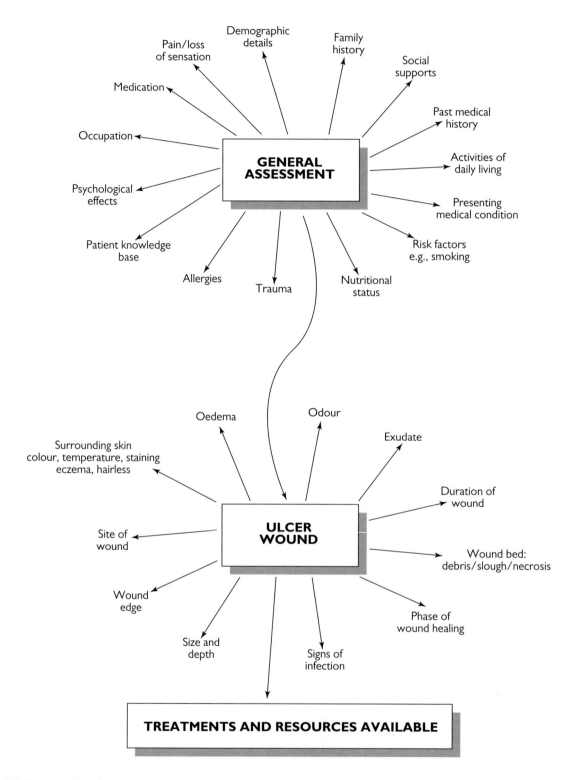

Fig. 5.9 Factors included in assessment.

Holistic assessment of a patient with a leg ulcer, using a standardized tool

While the leg ulcer assessment tool illustrated in Figure 5.10 is a useful prompt, ensuring that a full assessment is made, it is sometimes better to allow patients to tell their own story; by using their listening skills, and by prompting patients rather than asking specific questions, nurses can often elicit more information. The assessment tool needs to be used in conjunction with a full assessment of the activities involved in daily living.

Having a standardized tool does enable care to be provided with continuity. It is also useful for providing data required in audits measuring the effectiveness of patient management.

A chart defining the characteristics of ulcers of different aetiologies is presented in Chapter 2 (Table 2.3).

Risk factors

The risk factors are the same as those for other kinds of peripheral vascular disease. Here, psychological factors and self-neglect are prominent.

Past medical history

Apart from the general points mentioned above, the following have particular relevance for leg ulcers:

- venous insufficiency caused by previous DVT, phlebitis, varicose veins, pregnancy leading to venous hypertension
- Arterial disease, e.g. atherosclerosis leading to TIAs, CVA, coronary heart disease
- Diabetes
- Rheumatoid arthritis
- Skin malignancies
- Pelvic and abdominal surgery leading to increased risk of DVT
- Trauma leading to silent DVT
- Limited mobility
- Smoking.

Patient understanding

Evaluation of patients' own knowledge base in relation to the cause and prevention of ulceration is necessary in order to support their active involvement in their recovery.

Demographic influences

IQ does not appear to influence the incidence of leg ulceration, though Franks and Moffatt (1994) showed that it is higher in social class 3 than in 1. However, it needs to be recognized that the incidence may have more to do with financial constraints than with social class itself, and that retired people who identify themselves as belonging to social classes 1 and 2 may no longer have the financial means to protect themselves from the increased risk of ulceration that comes with age. This has a bearing on risk factors associated with leg ulceration; for example, the ability to afford properly fitting shoes if one is suffering from diabetic neuropathy.

ischaemia. The nurse needs to be aware of patients with mixed arterial and venous disease when considering compression bandaging, prescribing reduced compression in such patients only where the ABPI and history indicate that it is safe. Equally, calcification of vessels may give deceptively high readings—for example, in patients with diabetes or rheumatoid arthritis—and such patients need to be managed with caution and consideration, bearing in mind the possibility of microvascular disease.

Ankle pressures alone are not sufficient to detect impaired arterial circulation in patients with leg ulcers (Moffatt & Hare 1995); they need to be used in conjunction with a full medical and nursing history. More sophisticated investigation (e.g. angiography) may be required to confirm the diagnosis. Incorrect bandaging can cause damage severe enough to result in amputation or even death.

Ankle circumference

Measuring ankle circumference will help nurses to monitor oedema if present, and also to select the correct combination of pressure bandages for patients with venous ulceration only, where this is safe.

Oedema

Oedema is often present in patients with venous ulceration. However, it gives no indication as to the aetiology of the ulcer, as it can occur in any type. Oedema will inhibit the process of wound healing as it reduces the permeability of the healing tissues to oxygen. Causes include immobility, limb dependence, fixed ankle joint, cardiac or renal failure, hypoalbuminaemia and infection (Cullum & Roe 1995).

Moffatt (1994) suggests that over 50% of people over the age of 85 have some degree of arterial disease. This needs to be borne in mind when obtaining a differential diagnosis of an ulcer which gives all the outward signs of being of venous origin. Eliminating the possibility of mixed pathology enables the decision of whether or not to use compression, and to what strength, to be made safely.

Nutritional status

By itself obesity does not cause ulceration. However, when it is found alongside other risk factors—e.g. diabetes, hypertension or smoking—ulcers may be present and the obesity may impede wound healing. Where there is extreme pressure on the femoral vein due to rolls of fat pressing on the groin, blood flow may be occluded, reducing the supply of oxygen and nutrients required for the wound to heal. Equally, blood returning to the heart through the venous system may also be occluded owing to the pressure on the femoral vein, so allowing a build-up of metabolites and oedema that will hinder wound healing (Moffatt 1994).

To promote wound healing a patient needs adequate levels of protein, vitamins C and A, energy in the form of carbohydrates, and zinc and magnesium to assist in the production of collagen. Where there is anorexia or a heavy loss of protein in the wound exudate, healing will be compromised (Bryant 1994).

Medication

Steroids Patients taking steroids often have skin that is wafer-thin, making it vulnerable to trauma. In the process of wound healing, the inflammatory phase has an important role to play. As steroids dampen this down, they may also reduce the rate of wound healing.

Beta-blockers These cause peripheral vasoconstriction, and in the patient who is already arterially compromised there is an increased risk of leg ulceration.

Non-steroidal anti-inflammatory drugs The evidence is inconclusive as to the effect of these drugs on the healing wound. As they dampen down the inflammatory response there may be an effect on the inflammatory phase of wound healing.

Immunosuppressants, e.g. cyclophosphamide The patient who requires these drugs—for example following renal transplant—and who already has a vascular ulcer, is at increased risk of infection owing to the suppression of white cell production.

Antibiotics The skin is colonized by commensal bacteria. Overuse of antibiotics in patients with an ulcer containing commensal organisms can result in resistance. However, patients presenting with diabetes and an ulcer may be given antibiotics prophylactically as they are at greater risk of infection.

Assessment of pain

Ischaemic ulcers are often very painful, but any ulcer can cause pain. Pain is very subjective and personal, and therefore it is essential that patients be allowed to express the type and degree of pain they experience in their own way. Using a scale of 0–10, 0 being none and 10 being excruciating pain—the nurse will be able to assess how effectively treatment is controlling pain, making adjustments in analgesia in accordance with the drug prescriptions to suit the individual (Haywood 1994). Uncontrolled pain may also be a limiting factor in mobility, causing the patient to feel tired and sleepy to the point of exhaustion.

Mobility

The degree of mobility and amount of exercise undertaken by the patient requires assessment, as it often relates closely to the prognosis.

Exercise is crucial to the development of a collateral blood supply in the arterially compromised patient. For the patient with venous ulceration, Gardener and Fox (1991) illustrate the importance of the muscle pumps in the calf and foot in assisting the return of venous blood. Where this is hindered, metabolites and toxins will damage tissues, resulting in ulceration. An ankle joint that is fixed owing to arthritis will also compromise the integrity of the foot/calf muscle pumps. As long as there is ischaemia, the ability of wounds to heal will be affected.

Appearance of surrounding skin

Abnormal rubor or pallor in the supine or dependent limb, plus unusual skin temperature in a room that is set at a comfortable level, will indicate the presence of arterial disease. This will vary according to the ischaemic changes, but may range from a limb which is warm to the touch with dependent rubor and which becomes pale on elevation, to a leg which is cold and cyanosed.

In the presence of peripheral vascular disease and diabetic ulcers the leg may be unusually cold or warm, depending on the arterial status. Where vessels are occluded with thrombus or emboli the limb becomes cold. However, in the presence of the autonomic neuropathy that often develops in diabetic patients, vasodilatation may occur. Microvessels become engorged in a bid to bring oxygen to the tissues, thus producing a leg which is hot and oedematous. On elevation of the limb, colour is quickly lost, and the limb may take well over the normal 3 seconds to reperfuse.

In patients with rheumatoid arthritis and ulcers of other aetiology, skin colour and temperature usually remain unaffected, although brown pigmentation is a common feature in patients with venous insufficiency, owing to the presence of haemosiderin (the iron-containing part of haemoglobin) in the tissues.

Lipodermatosclerosis, eczema and a woody feel to the skin are often present (Table 2.3) (Cullum & Roe 1995).

Skin changes

Arterial disease
- shiny
- hairless skin
- sunset leg
- pain when walking

Venous disease
- haemosiderin staining
- oedematous
- purplish hue when dependent
- pain relieved by walking.

In the diabetic patient the skin on the feet may appear dry with cracks and fissures as a result of the loss of sweating caused by autonomic neuropathy. Motor neuropathy also causes atrophy of the small muscles of the foot, which will be characterized by deformities such as Charcot's joints and hallux valgus, hammer toes, claw toes and dropped foot arch. The resulting disproportion of body weight on the foot will alter the gait and may result in callus formation.

Sensation

This may be lost in the ischaemic or diabetic patient with ischaemic sensory neuropathy. Ulceration can arise where loss of sensation prevents a patient from recognizing that trauma is being caused to the foot—for example, through standing on foreign bodies or wearing ill-fitting shoes or tightly fitting socks that reduce blood flow in the already arterially compromised limb. A history of pins and needles or a sensation of walking on air that affects balance may be given.

Allergies

Many patients are sensitive to products containing lanolin, perfume or elastic (Table 13.16). Gaining knowledge before planning treatment may help to prevent reactions. Monitoring the progress of healing ulcers should alert the practitioner to any unknown allergies that may arise (Cameron 1990). The patient in Figure 2.9 (I) presented with an arterial ulcer, but developed a severe sensitivity reaction to the adhesive in a primary dressing.

Biopsy

Where ulcers continue to enlarge in spite of treatment, and present with raised rolled edges or a cauliflower appearance, biopsy may be required to provide a differential diagnosis for malignancy (Fig. 2.9 (G)).

Size of wounds

Measuring the area and depth of wounds will assist in monitoring the progress of wound healing. This can be achieved through photography with the use of a grid reference or tape measure. Liskay et al (1993) highlighted the importance of measurement and demonstrated the advantage of using a grid rather than a tape measure. Depth can be monitored by the insertion of a measured amount of cavity wound care product, such as Intrasite gel, or water via a syringe into the wound. Over a period of time the amounts of fluid inserted can be compared.

Perforating ulceration

Ulcers may track deep into the skin. Where an ulcer is not healing this should be investigated. Often the cause is a deep-seated infection or foreign body; for example, that caused by a chip of bone which has fragmented from osteomyelytic bone. X-ray may help to confirm the diagnosis.

Exudate

Heavy loss of protein-rich serous fluid may occur, reducing serum levels of albumin. Screening for hypoproteinaemia will help to confirm this, and steps will need to be taken to control the exudate and replace the albumin.

In the presence of infection the exudate may be offensive and purulent. Bleeding can arise, particularly where wounds are friable during the early stages of granulation and trauma is caused during management of dressings. Malignant ulcers may bleed or suppurate.

Screening for anaemia, particularly when varicose veins have ulcerated and haemorrhaged, will help to protect the patient from generalized malaise.

Psychosocial

Embarrassment caused by the odour from ulcers, along with attendant immobility and pain, may inhibit patients from enjoying normal social activities. They may become ulcer-dependent if they are lonely or depressed, because they look forward to the social contact with nursing staff. Addressing social issues through adequate assessment and intervention may help to improve patients' quality of life without the need for a wound. It is not unknown for patients to induce ulceration in order to maintain some kind of social contact.

Prevention is better than cure. The benefits of accurate assessment have been recognized by many leaders in the management of leg ulcers (Moffatt 1994, Cullum & Roe 1995, Ertl 1993, Vydelingum 1991, Jay 1989). These authors have evaluated the nurse's responsibility in holistically assessing patients with leg ulcers so that treatment plans can be effectively implemented, with the aim of reducing the prevalence of ulceration. The provision of an assessment tool from which to work will ensure that the treatment plan is based on a *complete* assessment.

For nurses to make a differential diagnosis it is essential that they have sound, research-based knowledge. The dissemination of this knowledge to other practitioners working in the field of leg ulceration will ensure that patients receive appropriate care, leading to the enjoyment of a better quality of life.

Professional responsibility has been outlined by Roe et al (1993) who believe that community nurses would benefit from further information on aetiology and the research-based management of patients with leg ulcers. It is hoped that the development of leg ulcer management courses, as well as local initiatives and national guidelines, will help to facilitate this.

REFERENCES

Barnhorst D A, Barner H B 1968 Prevalence of congenitally absent pedal pulses. New England Journal of Medicine 278: 268–275

Boore J 1996 Prescription for recovery. In: Research classic from the Royal College of Nursing. Scutari, London

Brearley S, Simms M, Shearman P 1992 Peripheral pulse palpation: an unreliable physical sign. Annals of the Royal College of Surgeons of England 74: 169–171

Bryant R 1994 Acute and chronic wounds: nursing management. Mosby, St Louis

Cameron J 1990 Patch testing for leg ulcer patients. Nursing Times 86(25): 63–64

Cameron J 1991 The consequences of incorrect Doppler ultrasound in differential diagnosis of venous and arterial lower limb pathologies. Nursing Standard 40: 25–27

Cullum N 1994 Nursing management of leg ulcers in the community. Liverpool University Press, Liverpool

Cullum N, Roe B 1995 Leg ulcer management. Scutari, London

Dimond B 1990 Legal aspects of nursing. Prentice-Hall, Englewood Cliffs, NJ

Ertl P 1991 Incidence and aetiology of leg ulcers. Professional Nurse 7(3): 190–194

Ertl P 1992 Looking beyond the ulcer itself. Assessment of leg ulcers. Professional Nurse 4: 258–262

Ertl P 1993 The multi benefits of accurate assessment. Professional Nurse 9(2): 139–144

Franks P, Moffatt C 1994 A pre-requisite underlying the treatment programme: risk factor associated with venous disease. Professional Nurse 9(9): 637–638, 640, 642

Gardener A M N, Fox J A 1991 In: Ertl P (ed) Incidence and aetiology of leg ulcers. Professional Nurse 7(3): 190–194

Hallett J W, Brewster D C, Darling R C 1995 Handbook of patient care in vascular surgery, 3rd edn. Little Brown, Boston

Haywood J 1994 Information—prescription against pain. Scutari, London

Jay P 1989 Assessing patients with leg ulcers in the community. Journal of Clinical Practice, Education and Management 33: 45–48

Liskay A M et al 1993 Comparison of two devices for wound measurement. Dermatology Nursing 5(6): 437–440

McIntosh J B 1979 Decision making on the district. Nursing Times 75(29): 77–80

Moffatt C 1994 Leg ulcer management—a colour guide series. Mosby, London

Moffatt C, Hare 1995 Graduated compression hosiery for venous ulceration. Journal of Wound Care 4(10): 459–462

Moffatt C et al 1994 Auditing a leg ulcer. Service 8(48): 52

Roe B et al 1993 Prevention and monitoring of chronic leg ulcers in the community. Journal of Clinical Nursing 5: 299–306

Smith F T C, Shearman C P, Simms M H, Gwunn B R 1994 Falsely elevated ankle pressures in severe leg ischaemia: the pole test—an alternative approach. European Journal of Vascular Surgery 8: 408–412

Taylor L M 1992 The incidence of perioperative myocardial interaction in general vascular surgery. Journal of Vascular Surgery 15: 52–61

Underwood M A 1983 Treatise on ulcers of the legs. Matthews, London

Vowden K R, Goulding V, Vowden P 1996 Hand-held Doppler assessment for peripheral arterial disease. Journal of Wound Care 5(3): 125–128

Vydelingum 1991 Assessing leg ulcers. Journal of Clinical Practice, Education and Management November 4(45): 24–26

FURTHER READING

Blank C A, Irwin G H 1990 Peripheral vascular disorders: assessment and intervention. Nursing Clinics of North America 25(4): 777–794

Gehring P E 1992 Perfecting the art of vascular assessment. Registered Nurse 55(1): 40–47

Hill S L 1991 Discharge planning for the vascular patient: where does care fit in? Journal of Vascular Nursing 9(3): 6–7

Implementation of nursing management

Caring for the patient with venous disorders

The aetiology and assessment of patients with venous disorders has already been discussed in some depth in Chapters 2 and 5. This chapter aims to address the nursing management of this patient group, highlighting the specific care required for disorders of different aetiology. It should not be forgotten, of course, that there are similarities in nursing practice and protocols whatever the disorder.

It is uncommon for superficial thrombophlebitis, venous ulcers or varicose veins to be life-threatening, although these three disorders of the venous system can be disfiguring and painful, and can have distressing effects on the quality of life. Deep vein thrombosis and pulmonary embolus, on the other hand, do present a significant threat to life.

Nurses are well placed to reduce the incidence of venous disorders and their complications. For example, appropriate management of cannulated patients undergoing intravenous infusion, cytotoxic therapy or investigations requiring the infusion of radiographic contrast should help to minimize the risk of *phlebitis*, although this can also result from trauma in patients already presenting with varicose veins and venous ulcers.

Prophylactic use of anticoagulants and anti-embolic hosiery where appropriate can help to prevent deep vein thrombosis in the surgical setting. Close observation of patients and a sensitive, early, relevant response to presenting signs and symptoms of deep venous thrombosis should contribute to a reduction in the risk of minor disorders developing into serious complications. Where deep vein thrombosis is recognized, appropriate treatment can be implemented at the earliest possible time, so reducing the risk of pulmonary embolus, chronic pulmonary hypertension or *post-thrombotic syndrome*, which may present at a later date in the form of venous stasis leading to venous ulceration or eczema.

Venous hypertension is a major contributor to the presentation of venous ulcers. Varicose veins may also contribute to ulceration. Varicosities may be congenital or acquired: in the latter case, occupations involving long periods of standing and abdominal pressure during pregnancy can be contributory factors. Fifteen per cent of the adult population are affected by varicose veins, and timely prophylaxis can forestall the development of varicose eczema and venous ulceration in later life.

Health promotion will help prevent the development of disease. For example, where patients are known to have venous hypertension and are at risk of developing venous leg ulcers, or where they have previously healed venous leg ulcers, explaining the relevance of wearing compression hosiery, of elevating the legs and of exercising may well reduce the incidence of ulceration. Figure 6.1 shows a device used to help patients put on compression hosiery.

PHLEBITIS

Signs and symptoms

Signs and symptoms are:

- pain, which is often at the site of cannulation

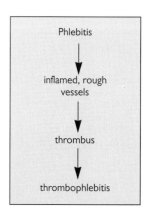

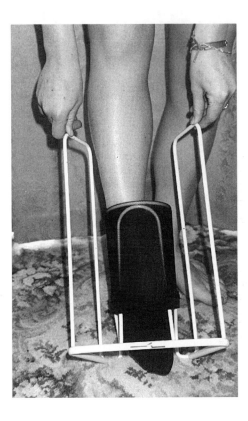

Fig. 6.1 Application of support hosiery with a Medi Valet stocking applicator.

- inflammation: redness, heat, swelling, reduction in mobility, pain, pus (N.B. Pus is not necessarily a sign of infection)
- a firm red streak following the path of the vein.

Treatment

Treatment includes:

- mandatory removal of cannula from site if present
- elevation of the affected limb
- non-steroidal anti-inflammatory medication for reduction of inflammation and pain relief
- antibiotics (possibly), should the patient present with a pyrexia or more than one sign of infection that is confirmed by culture of a wound swab
- warm compresses, which help to reduce oedema by stimulating the blood flow, or ice packs, which may be found soothing and aid the reduction of swelling, but need to be used with caution in the ischaemic patient.

Phlebitis is:

- pain
- heat
- redness
- swelling
- reduced mobility
- red streak tracking.

SUPERFICIAL THROMBOPHLEBITIS

If phlebitis remains unrecognized, *superficial thrombophlebitis* may develop. Thrombus is allowed to form because the vein has become inflamed and roughened, and the blood flow is therefore subject to turbulence. Thrombophlebitis presents when microorganisms such as staphylococci and streptococci proliferate in the lumen of the vessel around thrombus, and pus becomes trapped in pockets.

Because of the inaccessibility of the site, antibiotics are occasionally prevented from reaching the microorganisms, which may then circulate around the body, leading to septicaemia.

Treatment

- Treatment is as for phlebitis, with the addition of a small daily dose of aspirin, which has antithrombotic properties.
- Providing there is no evidence of deep vein thrombosis or ischaemia, compression will provide support to the veins, reducing the risk of long-term damage to the valves and therefore of venous hypertension.
- If there is any doubt as to the diagnosis, duplex scanning is performed to differentiate between superficial and deep vein thrombophlebitis or to identify the presence of suppurative thrombophlebitis.
- Should the thrombophlebitis develop to become suppurative, excision of the entire vein is required and systemic heparin is indicated.

Prophylactic nursing intervention

- Strict hand washing and aseptic techniques are mandatory when inserting a cannula.
- A cannula should be checked every 24 hours and resited every 72 hours in accordance with Department of Health guidelines or when there are signs of extravasation, inflammation or dislodgement of the cannula. Giving sets should be changed every 24 to 48 hours.
- Drugs and chemicals should be appropriately diluted prior to intravenous administration.
- The site of cannulation should be chosen with care.
- When piggybacked lines are no longer required, adaptors should be removed immediately.
- Hand washing is again mandatory prior to the administration of bolus infusions via an in situ cannula or as a secondary line.
- Cannula and continual infusion lines should be carefully handled and secured to prevent trauma and dislodgement.
- The patient should be monitored for low-grade pyrexia and signs of discomfort.
- In some centres GTN patches may be placed below the cannula in a bid to prolong the life of the site by enhancing venous dilatation and blood flow. This is contraindicated if the patient presents with a headache as a result of the procedure.

> How to prevent phlebitis from cannulae:
>
> - aseptic technique
> - check cannula every 24 hours
> - change giving sets every 48 hours
> - resite cannula every 72 hours
> - avoid irritable fluid concentrations
> - select sites carefully
> - remove adaptors, etc., when redundant
> - secure lines properly
> - watch for pyrexia, pain, etc.

DEEP VEIN THROMBOSIS (DVT)

Signs and symptoms

DVTs can be silent, especially in younger people who may have acquired them as a result of trauma; for example, rugby players who are kicked during play. They may present later in life with signs of venous hypertension such as leg ulcers.

A positive Homans' sign may only be present in as few as 20% of patients. It needs to be read with caution and in correlation with a full history, as trauma to a limb may equally cause pain on dorsiflexion.

Other signs and symptoms include:

- sudden, unilateral calf/thigh swelling
- tension in the tissues

- calf pain and a sensation of heaviness in the legs
- reduced mobility
- distended superficial veins.

Diagnostic testing

The following tests are used:

- venous duplex
- venogram.

Guidelines for the care of vascular patients with DVT

Observations

Immediate identification of a possible pulmonary embolus is essential. Vital signs should be recorded 4-hourly to permit monitoring of blood pressure, respiration, pulse and temperature. Oximetry may be indicated if the patient becomes breathless and presents with pulmonary embolus as a complication. Recording the calf and thigh circumference at regular intervals will allow accurate monitoring of the patient's progress.

Anticoagulation

Bed rest is essential during heparin therapy, which usually lasts for 5 days. A bolus dose of unfractionated heparin is followed by continuous infusion of the drug at 24 000–40 000 units per 24 hours, depending on patient size.

The heparin dose is monitored by reference to the activated partial thromboplastin time (APTT), which needs to be at least 1.5 times the patient's control value as recommended by the European Consensus Statement presented in 1992. An upper limit has not been agreed. It is recommended that blood levels should be measured midway between two injections.

Warfarin should be started during heparin infusion, as it usually takes about 2 or 3 days to reach a steady state. The International Normalized Ratio (INR) is the measure of warfarin activity. The dose should be titrated until the INR ranges between 2 and 3, and daily INR monitoring should be continued until the warfarin dose has been stabilized. The dose is adjusted according to the daily INR. The patient is discharged on warfarin for 2–6 months; warfarin for life is occasionally indicated where there has been repeated deep vein thrombosis.

The European Consensus Statement regarding the prevention of venous thrombosis states that:

> Low molecular weight heparins given subcutaneously have been shown to be as safe and effective as standard heparin therapy for the initial treatment of DVT when assessed for reduction of thrombus size by repeat venography. Preliminary results demonstrate that fixed dose body weight adjusted unmonitored low molecular weight heparins are as effective as adjusted dose intravenous standard heparin in the prevention of symptomatic recurrent venous thromboembolism during long-term follow-up.

The committee also concludes that thrombolytic therapy produces a more rapid and greater clot lysis in proximal DVT than unfractionated heparin, but it has not yet been established whether there is sufficient benefit to warrant its use.

Thrombectomy

This may be required for limb salvage.

Mobility

• The patient should be encouraged not to massage the leg, in the early days, as this increases the risk of throwing off a clot.

• Physiotherapy, passive leg exercises and the restoration of mobility should be delayed until the patient is fully heparinized.

• Once the patient is fully mobile, brisk walking, swimming, jogging and general exercise within his or her abilities will help to reduce the risk of venous hypertension by aiding the calf/foot muscle pump in promoting venous return.

• Leg elevation at 45° will help to reduce oedema, but this is best left until after the patient is fully warfarinized, in order to reduce the risk of pulmonary embolus.

Management of the patient with anti-embolic stockings

• No stockings should be worn until the patient is fully heparinized.

• Anti-embolic stockings should only be worn if no discomfort is experienced.

• Legs should be checked at least daily for signs of ischaemia or necrosis.

• Stockings should be removed each day to facilitate checks for any adverse reaction, washing of the legs and the application of emollient to keep the skin supple. On discharge patients may need to wear the stockings for several weeks in order to reduce recurrent oedema and to make themselves more comfortable.

• Long-term compression hosiery may be indicated to reduce the risk of venous hypertension and associated haemosiderin staining, lipodermatosclerosis or ulceration. However, after a DVT collateral superficial vessels may develop to recanalize the venous system, and the use of compression hosiery may result in occlusion of these new vessels, therefore exacerbating the situation.

• For long-term prophylactic use, stockings can be removed at bedtime, but should be put on again before the patient gets out of bed.

• Stockings should be hand washed using warm water. Compression hosiery should be renewed every 3 months.

> Anti-embolic stockings in DVT:
>
> • apply 23 mmHg pressure
> • should only be used when patient safely anticoagulated
> • necessitate daily checking of circulation
> • last about three months
> • are contraindicated if there is:
> — small vessel disease, diabetes, RA, etc.
> — ABPI < 0.8
> — claudication.

Contraindications to the wearing of anti-embolic stockings

Contraindications are as follows:

• DVT not anticoagulated

• microvascular disease as seen in diabetes and autoimmune disorders such as rheumatoid arthritis, polyarteritis nodosa, scleroderma, disseminated lupus erythematosus, temporal arteritis

• ABPI < 0.8

• history of arterial claudication or night/rest pain in legs or feet

• venous claudication resulting from occlusion of superficial venous collaterals by the compression hosiery.

Management of pain

Pain is managed by non-steroidal anti-inflammatory drugs unless there is a coexisting history of allergy or gastric ulceration. Mild codeine-based analgesics may be prescribed.

The prevention of deep vein thrombosis (DVT)

Inpatients are at increased risk of DVT because of immobility. Some are at particular risk because of:

• the nature of the patient, who may present with:
— obesity

— a past history of DVT or pulmonary embolus
— malignant disease or thrombophilic disorders
— pregnancy
• the nature of the admission and contributing factors such as:
— prolonged immobility, e.g. stroke
— pelvic, hip or knee surgery
— major trauma.

Three prophylactic measures are in common use, namely *anti-embolic stockings, subcutaneous low molecular weight heparin* and *intermittent pneumatic compression*. Many papers have proved the efficacy of each method separately, and using more than one is better still. The incidence of DVT in surgical patients is found to be reduced from 27% to 11% when stockings are worn and further reduced to 6% with additional heparin. Intermittent pneumatic compression also reduces the incidence from 27% to 18%, and in extreme cases all three methods can be used with benefit (Fig. 6.2). On cost-effectiveness grounds, one, two or three methods are used according to the risk.

Other prophylactic measures include stopping the combined oral contraceptive pill, preferably 6 weeks before an operation. The use of alternative measures for contraception during this time will, it is hoped, minimize the risk of pregnancy, which itself is a risk factor, especially when one considers that the projected 6 weeks' waiting period depends upon bed availability.

The use of low-dose warfarin or dextran as a prophylactic may be indicated.

Patient education

Patients should be made fully aware of the following:

• the effects of smoking

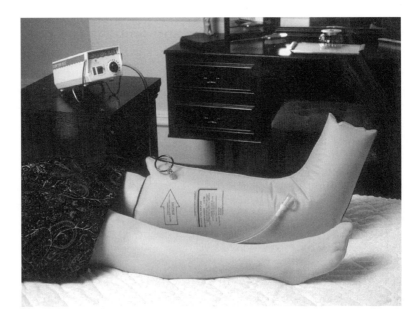

Fig. 6.2 Flotron intermittent pneumatic compression therapy used in the reduction of lymphoedema and to aid venous return.

- the effects of obesity
- the need to exercise
- the benefits of leg elevation, once they are fully heparinized, to aid venous return
- the importance of clothing that does not constrict the calves, thighs, groins, abdomen and waist, as this will impede venous return
- the benefits of compression hosiery, where appropriate, in aiding venous return and preventing future leg ulceration or recurrent DVTs
- instructions for medication. Where patients are discharged on warfarin, they should be aware of the need for regular INR checks, and of the importance of taking medication regularly as prescribed and of ensuring that repeat prescriptions are acquired prior to finishing a supply. They should be instructed to observe any unusual signs of bruising, swelling (haematoma) or excess bleeding, and to seek medical help immediately should these occur
- the need to discontinue birth-control pills containing oestrogen. Referral for family planning advice may be indicated.

PULMONARY EMBOLUS

The major source of pulmonary emboli is the legs. The embolus passes from the peripheral system into the pulmonary arterial tree via the right atrium and ventricle. If the embolus is large, death is almost instantaneous. However, it has been suggested that cardiac massage may help to break up the thrombus, and if the peripheral pulses and sufficient oxygenation can be restored quickly, the patient may survive; this, however, depends on the cardiac status, as there is a high risk of associated myocardial infarction.

Presenting signs

Presenting signs may include pleuritic chest pain, cough, wheezing, dyspnoea, hypoxia, respiration of less than 16 per minute, cyanosis, hypotension, cardiac arrhythmias, tachycardia and loss of consciousness. Pyrexia, chest infection and haemoptysis may also present.

Clinical investigations

Clinical investigations may include arterial blood gases, chest X-ray, isotope lung scan and pulmonary angiography, ECG and peak flow.

Treatment

Intervention to stabilize the critical incident will be a priority, and this may involve calling the resuscitation team. Oxygen will need to be administered immediately. Cardiac monitoring, oximetry blood pressure and pulse readings for rhythm, rate and volume will need to be maintained and recorded.

Patients and relatives will require reassurance and support to cope with the emotional distress associated with such a critical incident. Maintaining a controlled and calm environment will, therefore, help to generate a feeling of security.

Anticoagulants are administered as for patients with DVT. The dose of heparin may need to be increased in cases of pulmonary embolus in order to maintain the partial thromboplastin time at between 1.5 and 2.5, as heparin is utilized more quickly in this patient group. For patients with a large pulmonary embolus, intravenous heparin may be required for 5 to 10 days.

Thrombolytic therapy may include the use of agents such as tissue plasminogen activator (t-PA), urokinase and streptokinase in the dissolution of clots. A pul-

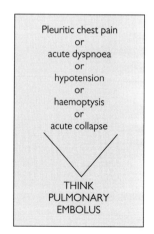

Pleuritic chest pain
or
acute dyspnoea
or
hypotension
or
haemoptysis
or
acute collapse

THINK
PULMONARY
EMBOLUS

monary catheter will be inserted under radiographic conditions. As well as acting as a route for the administration of thrombolytic agents, the catheter will permit serial angiography to be carried out in order to monitor the effectiveness of treatment.

Nursing guidelines

• Vital signs should be monitored and recorded, allowing staff to act in response to changing needs.

• Pulmonary assessment requires staff to monitor the colour of the patient, looking for signs of hypoxia, which may present as cyanosis, pallor or dyspnoea.

• The rate and level of respiration should be monitored, and any change in this, any nasal flaring or use of the accessory neck and shoulder muscles, should be noted.

• Oxygen therapy should be given as prescribed via a humidifier. Nasal cannulae are light and less obtrusive should longer-term oxygen be required. The decision on the percentage of oxygen to deliver during treatment will need to allow for any history of chronic obstructive airways disease.

Air embolism

All air needs to be removed from intravenous giving sets and syringes prior to the infusion of fluids, otherwise there is a risk of air embolism.

Nursing management

• Where the patient presents with an air embolism, placing them on their left side with the head of the bed tipped down will help to reduce the risk of this entering the right ventricle of the heart.

• At a later stage, if respiration is laboured, supporting the patient in an upright position may aid ventilation.

• The patient will need to be able to maintain adequate cardiac output. Checking pulse rate, rhythm and quality manually and using a cardiac monitor will alert the nurse to any deterioration so that medical support can be called for in good time.

• Nurses should check for distension of the neck veins, peripheral oedema and irregular ECG rhythms, which are indicative of pulmonary obstruction.

• The insertion of a Swan–Ganz catheter may be required in order to monitor the fluid load and pressure in the pulmonary artery. It is not uncommon for central venous pressure to remain elevated in a patient with a pulmonary embolism. This type of catheter may also be used to suck air out of the pulmonary artery.

• Prescribed medication should be administered to reduce the risk associated with cardiac arrhythmias, pulmonary hypertension, fluid overload, tachycardia and bronchial constriction. Digoxin should only be administered if the pulse rate rises above 60 beats per minute.

• Nurses should administer anticoagulation therapy as prescribed, observing any haemorrhaging, haemoptysis, tachycardia or hypotension.

• For the patient in shock, intravenous fluids will be administered and a fluid balance maintained, with care being taken not to overload the patient's circulatory system.

• Electrolytes and arterial blood gases will be monitored.

• Body temperature must be recorded to check the response to any signs of clinical infection.

• Pulmonary embolus is a sudden and critical incident which may result in extreme anxiety, as the patient experiences difficulty in breathing, chest pain and possible collapse. He or she will probably have undergone a great deal of medical and nursing intervention. One must explain the situation and actions taken to patients and their relatives, since reassurance will help to reduce anxiety and enable patients to participate in their care.

- A calm and quiet environment should be maintained.
- Analgesia should be administered as prescribed and its effectiveness monitored, with adjustments being made as needed.
- Patients should be positioned as comfortably in bed as possible.
- Patients' internal and external environment should be conducive to sleep, enabling them to obtain the rest they need to aid recovery.
- Patients should have a sound knowledge and understanding of prophylactic measures implemented to reduce the risks associated with deep vein thrombosis and pulmonary embolism; for example, doing passive leg exercises, not crossing the legs, deep breathing, wearing anti-embolic stockings once fully warfarinized, taking anticoagulation therapy as prescribed and ensuring that regular INR screening is maintained.
- Intermittent pneumatic compression of the veins in the lower limbs may help to reduce the risk of thrombus formation associated with venous stasis.
- Patients should be mobilized as soon as possible to reduce venous stasis and the risk of further emboli developing.
- Bed rest should be maintained until the patient is stabilized.
- The risk of pressure sore development should be assessed, and action taken to prevent this.
- Nutrition should be maintained.
- Assistance should be given with hygiene and mouth care as required.
- Patients should be assisted with micturition and elimination as required. Catheterization may be needed to ensure that the fluid balance is strictly maintained.
- Vital signs should be carefully monitored.

Inferior vena cava filter

Where anticoagulation therapy is contraindicated, it may be possible to insert a filter into the inferior vena cava to reduce the risk of pulmonary embolism.

NURSING MANAGEMENT OF PATIENTS WHO DEVELOP VARICOSE VEINS

The purpose of early treatment of varicose veins is to reduce the risks of stasis oedema, pain, ulceration and disfigurement associated with venous incompetence. To achieve this an initial conservative programme will address issues such as weight control, exercise, elevation, and compression hosiery if it is not contraindicated (see Ch. 5).

Compression hosiery

This can be acquired on prescription. The patient should be fitted to ensure that the appropriate size and level of compression is achieved, as determined by Stemmer's work (Stemmer et al 1980). 23 mmHg compression at the ankle may be sufficient to give the necessary level of support. Elderly patients may have difficulty in putting

Treatment of varicose veins:

- ligation of saphenofemoral junction
- avulsion (destruction) of the sites of the perforators
- stripping of the saphenous vein
- cryosurgery.

on stockings, and therefore a stocking applicator is recommended, e.g. Medi Valet (Fig. 6.1).

Teaching the patient to care for the stockings and making them aware of the importance of the components of a conservative management programme will improve compliance.

Elevation

When the ankle is placed at 45° above the level of the heart, gravity will aid venous return, so reducing venous hypertension: 'toes above nose'. Not all patients will be able to achieve this owing to coexisting arthritis, but elevation of the foot of the bed will enable patients to enjoy the same benefits while keeping the mattress flat.

Exercise

Any foot or leg movement which works the foot/calf muscle pump will aid venous return. Walking, swimming and cycling are highly recommended activities, providing they are within the capabilities of the patient.

Diuretics

Diuretics are only appropriate where other conditions coexist, e.g. heart failure. They will otherwise fail to reduce ankle oedema in the presence of venous insufficiency.

SCLEROTHERAPY

Sclerotherapy is used either in isolation or where stripping or ligation of the veins has failed to resolve the problem completely. It is also useful for treating large *telangiectases* (prominent spider-like venules).

Sclerotherapy is contraindicated if there is a past history of DVT, if there is local infection, or if veins present in the lower third of the leg (owing to the pain this would cause and the impossibility of achieving sufficient compression over the foot).

The sclerosant is usually sodium tetradecyl sulphate. The perforators and other prominent veins are identified and mapped out whilst the patient is standing. The patient is then laid supine while the sclerosant is infused. The object is to destroy the endothelium.

By its very nature, the sclerosing agent is irritant, so to feel some burning, itching or pain and to see rubor or local swelling is usual. Some thrombus formation is inevitable, but with elevation and compression this is minimal.

The compression is left for 1–3 weeks. Early mobilization is recommended to clear any residual sclerosant from the deep venous system.

The advantages of this treatment are that no anaesthetic is required. The patient is mobilized at the earliest possible time and treatment can be performed on a day-case basis, so reducing costs. The disadvantages are a high potential for allergic rashes, a continuing sensation of burning pain, local skin necrosis and thrombophlebitis. There is also a high risk of early collateral formation.

Nursing management

Preprocedure for sclerotherapy is as follows:

- Check for a history of allergy.
- Ensure that antiplatelet drugs, e.g. aspirin, are stopped a week prior to procedure.
- Check that patients with heart valve lesions have penicillin cover.

- Ensure that patients are able to give informed consent.
- Give information about bruising, pigmentation and the possible development of small nodules.

SURGERY FOR VARICOSE VEINS

Surgery for varicose veins may involve:

- saphenofemoral (or saphenopopliteal) ligation
- multiple avulsions of perforators
- stripping of the long saphenous vein.

Pre-operatively the geography of the veins is mapped out whilst the legs are dependent, using venous duplex.

It is usual to perform ligation plus multiple avulsions or all three procedures. It has been shown that to perform all three leads to better, longer-lasting results (Sarin & Scurr 1994). Duplexing and clinical assessment 21 months after surgery has demonstrated that there are fewer persisting incompetent veins after stripping, slower refilling times, less recurrence and increased patient satisfaction with the result.

The junction where the proximal end of the saphenous vein enters the femoral vein is identified and ligated. In the case of the short saphenous vein this is the junction with the popliteal vein behind the knee.

Stripping of the long saphenous vein is possible between the groin and the knee. During the stripping procedure, a wire is inserted into the vein in the groin and fed down towards the knee, at which point it is exposed via a second incision. A cap is secured onto the protruding end of the wire and it is then drawn back through the lumen of the vein, stripping the vein from the perforators.

Avulsions of perforators

Venous duplex studies are now used in preference to clinical assessment alone to identify the position of perforators whilst the patient is standing. Sometimes a hand-held Doppler is sufficient.

Under a general anaesthetic, small incisions are made over the underlying perforators, which are tied off, leaving the intervening lengths of vein intact.

Other methods of dealing with veins include *cryosurgery*, which involves the use of a liquid-nitrogen-cooled probe at the points where the perforators meet the saphenous veins (Garde 1994), or *ambulatory phlebectomy* (Cohn et al 1995), during which veins are removed under local anaesthetic with the leg dependent. These are clinic (outpatient) procedures which avoid the use of theatre time and seem to give good cosmetic results.

Postoperatively, the leg is immediately elevated and firmly bandaged, the compression being used to establish haemostasis.

Elevation continues for 24 hours, after which the patient is actively mobilized, with the compression remaining in place all day for 5 days. Support stockings can be removed after the first night at bedtime, but should be replaced before the patient gets out of bed in the morning.

Recurrent varicose veins can be a nuisance for patients, and work is being carried out in some centres to prevent these. The use of *laparoscopic surgery* to clip the ovarian vein can improve this situation.

Complications of venous surgery include haematoma formation, which may be largely averted by prompt and efficient bandaging with adhesive strapping, and damage to the saphenous nerve, resulting in patchy anaesthesia and pain. In 2% of cases DVT has occurred. Later complications include lymphoedema due to damage to perivenous lymphatics, discoloration of the skin due to haemosiderin deposition after heavy bruising, and residual or recurrent varicose veins.

Complications of varicose vein surgery:

- bruising
- haemorrhage at incision site
- pain
- patchy numbness
- DVT

and later:

- discoloration of the skin
- recurrent veins
- lymphoedema.

NURSING MANAGEMENT OF PATIENTS UNDERGOING VENOUS SURGERY

It is important that patients are given careful counselling so that they know what to expect after the operation. In one study 65.8% of patients perceived that within 2 weeks they had developed a complication, usually bruising, pain or numbness (Mackay et al 1995). Of the patients who consulted their general practitioners about these complications, half required reassurance only. The conclusion drawn in this study was that good preparation and peri-operative communication involving the use of comprehensive patient leaflets would have pre-empted many of the problems or reduced their significance to the patient.

Preparation for venous surgery

- Check the past medical history and everyday activities.
- Check that patients with heart valve lesions have penicillin cover.
- Ensure that the patient is able to give informed consent.
- Give information about bruising and the need for postoperative elevation, compression and exercise.

Postoperative procedures

- Monitor, record and respond to any deterioration in vital signs.
- Check dressing regularly for haemorrhage. Elevation or direct pressure may be required to bring this under control.
- Check foot pulses and motor function of limbs, especially where direct pressure has been applied in order to reduce haemorrhage.
- Maintain compression for 1–2 weeks postoperatively.

The skin closures are usually removed around the 7th to 10th postoperative day.

Advising the patient to elevate the limb when sitting will help to reduce the risk of bruising and oedema formation. Standing for long periods of time should be discouraged and walking as far as possible each day for at least 30 minutes should be encouraged. Any discomfort should be controlled using mild analgesic medication, as prescribed.

If the patient is to be discharged on the same day, the theatre bandages are usually taken down in hospital and anti-embolic stockings supplied. The patient should be asked to sleep in anti-embolic stockings on the first night, but after this he or she can remove the stockings at bedtime, replacing them before getting out of bed in the morning. Stockings should be worn for 6 postoperative weeks to reduce the risk of thrombus formation.

> Anti-embolic stockings are useful after varicose vein surgery and provide 14 mmHg pressure.

Anti-embolic stockings provide 14 mmHg pressure at the ankle and caution needs to be used to ensure that there is sufficient arterial perfusion to support this (ABPI > 0.7).

In order to avoid a recurrence of varicose veins, long-term management should include advice to wear support hosiery, to avoid standing or sitting with crossed legs, and to elevate the legs whenever possible.

VENOUS HYPERTENSION

Venous hypertension may occur as a complication of phlebitis, DVT, pulmonary embolus, varicose veins, and any situation which puts pressure on the central venous system, such as pelvic and hip surgery, tumour, pregnancy, obesity, occupations which involve prolonged standing, and congenital absence of valves. These situations result in high levels of venous pressure and backflow which damages the valves.

After thrombosis, if recanalization does not occur, collateral vessels form around the site of occlusion. In either case there will be a detrimental effect on venous return achieved by the foot/calf muscle pump action, as there are no valves in the vessels. This can result in venous claudication, which may be experienced as a 'bursting sensation', relieved by elevation of the limbs. In this respect it differs from arterial claudication.

The high pressures may also lead to haemosiderin staining, lipodermatosclerosis and ulceration, as discussed in Chapter 2.

VENOUS GANGRENE

Should the deep veins become severely occluded with thrombus and be lacking in a sufficient collateral supply to aid venous return, venous hypertension may become severe, leading to damage of the microcirculation in line with the white cell trapping theory and fibrin cuff theory (Ch. 2). This will prevent diffusion of nutrients, gases and waste products, and may occasionally lead to venous gangrene.

REFERENCES

Cohn M et al 1995 Ambulatory phlebectomy using the tumescent technique for local anaesthesia. Dermatologic Surgery 21(4): 315–318

Garde C 1994 Cryosurgery of varicose veins. Journal of Dermatologic Surgery and Oncology 20(1): 56–58

Mackay D C et al 1995 The early morbidity of varicose vein surgery. Journal of the Royal Naval Medical Service 81(1): 42–46

Sarin S, Scurr J 1994 Stripping of the long saphenous vein in the treatment of primary varicose veins. British Journal of Surgery 81(10): 1455–1458

Stemmer R et al 1980 Compression treatment of the lower extremities, particularly with compression stockings. The Dermatologist 31: 355–365

FURTHER READING

Drugs and Therapeutics Bulletin 1992 30(3)

Laing W 1992 Chronic venous diseases of the leg. (Studies of current health problems 108.) OHE, London

Robins M 1992 Epidemiologically based needs assessment. Report: varicose vein treatments. (Provisional version, commissioned by the NHS Management Executive)

Royal College of Nursing 1993 Who's doing the leg work? The real benefits of compression hosiery (RCN clinical issue series 43). RCN, London (Video production)

CHAPTER 7

Caring for the patient with leg ulcers

Many authoritative texts have been written on wound care and leg ulcer management. This chapter serves only to touch on *some* of the management criteria involved in caring for the patient with a leg ulcer.

The epidemiology and assessment of patients with vascular ulcers have been discussed in previous chapters. The nursing management of ulcers and prevention of reulceration will now be addressed. Regardless of the aetiology some of the interventions will be the same, but it must be remembered that each case needs to be managed to meet the needs of the individual patient.

Management of leg ulcers aims to:

- *improve quality of life*
- *reduce pain*
- *correct underlying causes by:*
  — reducing venous incompetence by aiding venous return through the use of compression hosiery where this is safe to do so
  — enhancing arterial blood flow
  — reducing inflammation
  — ensuring there is sufficient nutritional support to promote wound healing
- *create an optimum environment for wound healing at the wound site by*:
  — choosing primary dressings appropriately
  — ensuring cleansing is thorough and follows a safe technique
  — ensuring there is a compatible environment for wound healing
- *address holistically factors contributing to ulceration, for example:*
  — poor mobility
  — malnutrition
  — adverse social environment
  — smoking habits
  — obesity
  — inadequate diabetic control
  — lifestyle issues
- *Prevent:*
  — social isolation and loss of self-esteem
  — pain
  — loss of mobility and independence
  — wound infection
  — breakdown of wound and surrounding skin
  — medicament dermatitis
  — stasis oedema
  — reulceration once ulcer is healed.

ASSESSMENT

This should take account of general patient information and specific ulcer-related factors to allow accurate differential diagnosis and appropriate holistic management, in order to promote healing and enhance the patient's quality of life.

Assessment of patients with leg ulcers should always include:

- patient-related factors
- ulcer-related factors
- resources available

so permitting the provision of holistic care.

General patient information required

- Demographic details, family history and occupation or pastimes.
- Previous medical history. Consideration needs to be given to a history which includes coronary heart disease, transient ischaemic attacks, stroke, hypertension, diabetes mellitus, collagen disorders, autoimmune disorders, trauma, deep vein thrombosis, varicose veins and previous ulceration.
- Presenting signs and symptoms. These may include position of ulcer, shape of ulcer, abnormal haematology, biochemistry and microbiology, raised blood sugar levels, neuropathic changes, bone deformities, changes in cardiovascular status, presence of varicose veins and state of surrounding skin (which may include stasis oedema, colour of limb, state of toenails and foot deformities, presence of lipodermatosclerosis, atrophie blanche, capillary flare shiny hairless skin, variable skin temperature gradient in limbs).
- Assessment of the pain cascade, identifying type of pain, time of pain (claudication, pain at rest, night pain, venous claudication), duration, activities and the position of the limb which reduces pain, and the effectiveness of analgesics.
- Results of investigations such as blood and urine screening, and resting pressure index.
- Radiological investigations, including straight X-ray to determine the presence of foreign bodies such as calcified debris, bony changes of osteomyelitis, splinters, etc.; venography to identify the cause of venous hypertension; arteriography to assess the arterial status and demonstrate the presence of any occlusive disease.
- Ankle brachial pressure index (normal = 0.8–1.2). Less than 0.8 indicates ischaemia; elevation above 1.2 may indicate calcification of vessels or oedema, resulting in falsely elevated pressure masking underlying ischaemia. Figure 7.1 shows a district nurse undertaking Doppler assessment in a patient's home.

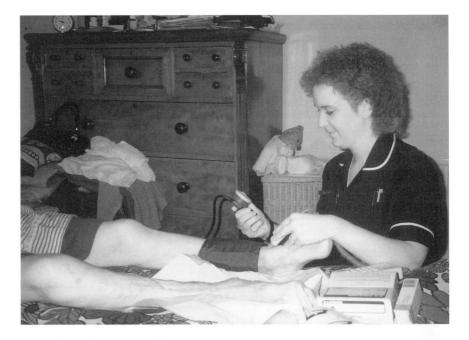

Fig. 7.1 A district nurse assessing ABPI on a patient at home.

- Biopsy to eliminate malignant ulceration.
- Allergies/sensitivity to previous treatments.
- Level of mobility.
- Nutritional status.
- Patient's level of understanding.

Ulcer-related information

Ulcer-related information includes stage of wound healing, duration of ulceration, status of wound bed, position of ulcer, size, shape, exudate, odour, clinical signs of infection, local pain, response to previous treatments, and what treatment options are available within the primary and secondary care sector.

Once a differential diagnosis has been established, as outlined in Chapter 5, nursing management can be planned.

Nursing goals

The ulcer will have an impact on the patient's daily activities, and this will need to be addressed together with the management of the ulcer.

It is not always possible to heal leg ulcers, but it is important to aim to maximize the patient's quality of life, either by ameliorating the presenting situation or taking prophylactic measures to reduce recurrence.

Informed patient consent to treatment should always be included in *nursing documentation.*

The nursing plan

The plan serves to identify potential problems which may arise in patients presenting with vascular ulcers of any aetiology, and therefore the nurse needs to be discriminating when completing individual patient care plans (Table 7.1).

Table 7.1 Patient care plan

Problem/need	Goal	Intervention
Anxiety	Enhance patient's understanding in order to reassure him/her and reduce anxiety	Listen and talk to the patient
		Reinforce emotional support
		Explain procedures before implementing them
Pain	Ensure patient is free from pain	Assess pain position, type, duration, exacerbating factors, exercise tolerance, presence of pain at night
		Give analgesic medication regularly as prescribed
		Monitor effectiveness of analgesia
		In the presence of ischaemic pain, place the limb in a dependent position, or elevate the head of the bed to aid perfusion

Cont'd

Table 7.1 Patient care plan (cont'd)

Problem/need	Goal	Intervention
Mobility is restricted by pain, stasis, oedema or fixed arthritic ankle joints	Enable patient to maximize mobility	Assess level of mobility
		Within patient limits, encourage mobilization of lower limbs
		Promote flexion of the ankle and movement of the foot/calf muscle pump
		Reduce pain in order to promote mobility
		Ensure patient has appropriate footwear
		Refer for physiotherapy as appropriate and ensure patient is able to use any mobility aids safely
Sleep is disturbed by pain	Improve quality of sleep, ensuring the patient receives sufficient rest	Provide an environment suited to the patient's individual needs
		Ensure medication to relieve pain and to enhance sleep is administered
		Relieve pressure from bedding using bed cradle
Patient is constipated (this may be a result of compounds used in analgesic medication, discomfort in getting to the toilet or coexisting bowel disorder)	Minimize difficulty in elimination	Administer medication to relieve constipation, as prescribed
		Ensure the patient is able to get to the toilet without pain
		High roughage diet
Patient needs to maintain personal hygiene	Ensure patient is able to maintain personal hygiene	Assist with hygiene as required
Communication	The patient is able to express needs and anxieties	Give the patient opportunity to talk
		Listen to the patient and respond sensitively to his/her communication
The patient lacks knowledge	Enable patient to verbalize or demonstrate understanding of given information	Explain to the patient using jargon-free language
	Ensure patient is able to give informed consent regarding treatment	Information should include: — why the patient has a leg ulcer — what can be done to promote healing — details on treatments undertaken — how patient can prevent re-ulceration
The patient is malnourished and presents with a low serum albumin owing to heavy serous exudate loss	Improve patient's nutritional status	Ensure that patient is able to take a high-calorie diet rich in protein, zinc, magnesium and vitamins C, D and A

Cont'd

Table 7.1 Patient care plan (cont'd)

Problem/need	Goal	Intervention
Patient is socially isolated owing to difficulty in mobilizing, and to offensive odour from wound	Enable patient to interact socially Eliminate any embarrassing odour	Control odour in wound management and provide odour-absorbing wound-care products
Stasis oedema is exacerbating leg ulceration and slowing the healing process	Reduce oedema	Elevate limb if there is no ischaemia to aid venous return Encourage active leg exercise to stimulate foot/calf muscle pump Apply intermittent compression therapy as prescribed Apply compression bandages if there is no ischaemic contraindication
The patient has a venous leg ulcer or stasis venous eczema	Promote healing Keep ulcer free from infection Improve quality of life	Follow wound care protocol when managing wounds Implement infection-control protocol when managing leg ulcers Change dressing if there is exudate strikethrough to reduce the risk of bacteria entering the wound and to enhance patient comfort Assess wound bed and stage of healing when selecting dressing Record and acknowledge any known allergies to dressing products when selecting an appropriate leg ulcer dressing Record ankle circumference and ABPI Apply compression accordingly

THE PREVENTION OF 'DIABETIC FOOT' ULCERS

Diabetic foot ulcers are common. The prevalence is 2% of diabetics at any one time. Sadly, 25% of diabetics go on to become amputees.

Assessment

Full vascular assessment is undertaken as previously described. Ischaemia is less likely to be associated with pain than in the other arteriopathies because of the sensory neuropathy.

Sensation can be tested with light touch and a tuning fork. An electrical stimulation device, which is quantitative and may detect the degree of loss of sensation, is available. Abnormal gait may indicate motor neuropathy.

Checking the skin for abnormal temperature, dryness, callus and fissures will help to identify diabetic foot. Pressures under the foot may be measured with a pedobarograph in specialized centres, but observation of the sole and the heel of the shoes for wear will give some indication of abnormal gait.

Simple ward urinalysis or ward blood glucose testing may demonstrate high sugar levels. However, average blood sugar over a period of time may be measured more accurately with the glycosylated haemoglobin test (HbA1$_c$). Persistent hyperglycaemia leads to defective collagen synthesis, which will affect the integrity of the skin.

Small vessel disease is a feature of diabetic disease. An estimate of capillary circulation can be made by compressing and releasing a toe; blanching should recover within 3 seconds. A loss of Doppler signal on elevation of the limb will indicate calcification of large vessels.

Management

Prevention can be achieved by:

- good control of blood sugar
- avoidance of trauma
- not walking barefooted
- checking feet for calluses, cracks and inflammation
- wearing supportive, properly fitting footwear
- taking care when using hot-water bottles and having a hot bath
- not soaking for too long in the bath to reduce the risk of softening the skin and allowing infection to enter
- visiting a chiropodist/podiatrist at regular intervals
- not using corn remedies
- not cutting toenails too short
- daily use of emollients to keep the skin supple
- reducing heel strike by inserting the kind of dynamic insoles found in high-quality trainers.

WOUND MANAGEMENT GUIDELINES FOR PATIENTS WITH LEG ULCERS (Example)

- The practitioner should have a sound research-based knowledge of the aetiology of wound healing and products suitable for each type of wound at each of the four stages of wound healing.
- Turner's characteristics of the ideal dressing should be taken into consideration when selecting products (Box 7.1).
- Each clinical area will be responsible for providing information on new research and available products.
- The nurse should be able to demonstrate knowledge and skills in the application of wound care products, including retention and compression bandages.
- Wound management will be approached holistically, ensuring the best possible lifestyle, nutrition and level of mobility for promoting wound healing.
- Each wound will be assessed using the standardized leg ulcer assessment form.
- The wound will be mapped out or photographed on initial assessment and at each review, which should be at least every 2–4 weeks.

Holistic assessment will allow safe holistic care.

■ BOX 7.1

Turner's 19 characteristics of an ideal dressing
- maintains a moist environment
- allows gaseous exchange—O_2, CO_2, water vapour
- maintains thermal insulation
- provides mechanical protection
- conformable and mouldable (e.g. to heels, sacrum)
- needs infrequent changing
- impermeable to microorganisms (in both directions)
- free from particulate contamination
- non-adherent
- safe to use (non-toxic, non-allergenic, non-sensitizing)
- acceptable to the patient
- cost-effective
- highly absorbent
- able to carry medicaments, e.g. antiseptics
- able to allow monitoring of a wound (e.g. transparent dressings)
- capable of standardization and evaluation
- non-inflammable
- able to be sterilized
- available in the primary and secondary care sectors in a suitable range of sizes
  (Morgan 1994)

- Each area will have a resource for illustration of ulcers.
- Dietary supplements will be given as needed to ensure sufficient intake of protein, calories, iron, vitamins A, D and C, zinc and magnesium.
- Help with mobility will be arranged as needed.
- Patient compliance will be best secured by:
  — considering the patient's lifestyle and special needs
  — informing patients, verbally and in printed form, about the causes of ulceration and reasons for management strategies
  — promoting active involvement in wound healing
  — giving patients at home contact telephone numbers for out-of-hours times should their wounds become uncomfortable
  — giving patients at risk of ulceration written information relating to the care of compression hosiery if there is a venous aetiology and to appropriate preventative treatment whatever the aetiology.
- Dressings should be left intact for as long as possible to avoid disturbing the wound.
- Where strikethrough presents in secondary dressings, the primary dressing needs to be managed to ensure that there is no risk to the skin surrounding the wound as a result of excoriation from exudate or entry of bacteria through a moist environment.
- Clean technique should be employed in washing the leg ulcer to remove all excess exudate, debris and wound care products from the previous dressing.
- The leg should be washed at each dressing change. Tap water and emollients can be used.
- Can be irrigated with warmed bags of saline where available; the quantity will depend on the ulcer size.
- All loose devitalized tissue should be removed, using forceps if necessary.

- Legs should not be left to soak and become soggy.
- Aseptic technique should be employed when re-applying the dressing.
- Local infection control will help to minimize the risk of clinical infection.
- Wounds should be kept warm, as once the temperature drops to below 37°C wound healing will be delayed by at least 4 hours (Miller 1994). It is suggested that, in the presence of bilateral ulceration, dressings should be removed from one ulcer at a time.
- It is recommended that dressings should be removed only when they can be immediately replaced.
- Assessment of pain at each dressing change will help the nurse to ensure that adequate pain relief is given prior to dressing and to gauge the right level of analgesic to prescribe between dressings.
- Keeping wounds in a moist warm environment will help to prevent the irritation of nerve endings, thereby reducing pain.
- Where wounds are caused by venous hypertension, legs should be elevated to reduce oedema and to aid venous return and the diffusion of nutrients and waste products to and from the tissues, which can be inhibited by oedema.
- Should the ulcer be arterial in origin, elevation of the head of the bed will aid arterial perfusion of the lower limbs, so enhancing diffusion of essential nutrients and oxygen to the tissues.
- Documentation must be maintained at each patient contact.
- Holistic evaluation of the patient's needs will ensure that care is responsive and adaptive.

MANAGEMENT GUIDELINES FOR INFECTION CONTROL IN ULCER CLINICS (Example)

- Wound swabs may be taken on the first assessment or if they are clinically indicated, bearing in mind the courier time for transportation to the laboratory. The swab is normally taken prior to cleansing; however, where much debris and wound care products such as iodine-based dressings remain on the wound, it may not be possible to achieve this. The important factor is to swab as deeply as possible into the wound. If the wound is dry, dampening the swab will enhance the collection of microorganisms. It is preferable to collect swabs from healthy wound tissue when this is present, rather than from areas of slough or necrosis. If there is a large amount of pus, this can be collected in a syringe (Wilson 1995).
- Systemic antibiotic therapy is only indicated where there are clinical signs of infection supported by microbiology sensitivity results.
- In the presence of methicillin-resistant *Staphylococcus aureus* (MRSA), topical Bactroban (mupirocin) may be prescribed for small wounds. This can be applied up to three times a day and is recommended for use up to 10 days only at any one time. However, where patients present with venous leg ulcers, consideration needs to be given to the most cost-effective form of treatment. It may be considered more appropriate to apply Bactroban only at each dressing change in order to sustain compression over a few days. Continued use of compression will be more effective in treating the underlying venous pathology which is resulting in ulceration. As the ulcers heal, the MRSA is likely to be eradicated.
- Treatment of MRSA in any other part of the body requires daily conventional therapy as per local protocols.

- Where there are clinical signs of infection systemic antibiotics should be administered according to the patient's prescription.
- For patients with MRSA, three clear swabs are required to determine that the microorganism has been eradicated. Normal swabbing protocols should be adhered to.
- According to the wound care protocol, ulcers should be throughly cleansed. It is not necessary to use Hibiscrub to wash ulcers that are colonized/infected with MRSA; they can be cleansed with warm tap water and a selected emollient in the usual fashion. For arterial ulcers, using warmed saline to irrigate the ulcers may be the best way of reducing the risk of introducing systemic infection.
- To reduce the risk of infection at each dressing change, all debris, including wound care products, exudate and loose slough/necrotic tissue, should be cleansed away.
- Clean wound care management should be implemented for cleansing, but an aseptic technique should be used to apply wound care products to the wound.
- Should exudate strike through the outer layer of dressings, these should be covered with a dry dressing if they cannot be changed immediately, in order to reduce the risk of microorganisms penetrating the wound. The whole dressing should then be changed at the earliest possible time.
- Where patients present with a clinical infection, they should be treated with the appropriate antibiotic. For outpatients with MRSA, it is preferable to treat them with sensitivity within their own home rather than bringing them into a clinic.
- Where outpatients with MRSA are required to attend the clinic in an ambulance, the ambulance service should be informed and local policy adhered to.
- It is preferable to attend to patients with MRSA at the end of a clinic if possible.
- Local infection controls should be implemented when managing patients with any kind of infection, including MRSA.
- Disposable, non-sterile aprons and gloves must be changed between patients. Hands must be washed between patients. Gloves may be removed after the application of the wool layer during bandaging.
- Doppler probes should be cleaned between the assessment of each patient. In order to protect the sensitive electrode at the end of the probe, it is important not to dunk it into a bowl of water. Where debris remain on the probe, this can be removed with a damp cloth prior to wiping with an alcohol-impregnated swab.
- For the assessment of ABPI, if the pulse point is within a leg ulcer the Doppler can be applied to the wound bed, which may be protected with a 90% water-based product, e.g. Geliperm Wet. (This product has been recognized as being safe for this practice by the Dressings Registration Authority.)
- Sphygmomanometer cuffs should be protected from wound exudate by placing clingfilm or a protective dressing over ulcerated areas in the region of pulse points at the ankle. They should be cleaned in accordance with the manufacturer's recommendations should they become soiled.
- Emollients should preferably be used for individual patients (i.e. each patient brings his or her own tub to each clinic). If this is not possible, disposable spatulae should be used to remove emollient from the tub.
- If heavily contaminated, bandage scissors must be washed and cleaned with 70% alcohol between patients. If they are not heavily contaminated, it is satisfactory to use a 70% alcohol wipe only. They should always be washed and wiped with 70% alcohol at the end of the clinic. Several pairs of scissors should be kept in each clinical area.

- Removal of skin scales should be carried out between patients and at the end of the clinical session, using the brush and pan provided.
- All surfaces should be washed with detergent and dried at the end of the clinic. Between patients, if there is no spillage, the sheet and/or the blue tissue roll lining should be changed.
- Each clinic should ensure that contaminated water from buckets is disposed of in a dedicated sink or sluice and that it is washed and dried thoroughly at the end of each session.
- Foot buckets must be washed with detergent and dried thoroughly. (Plastic liners may be used for individual patients.) Even if plastic liners are used, buckets should still be washed and *dried* between patients. There should be sufficient bowls/buckets for each patient attending the clinic session.
- At the end of the clinic, bowls should be washed with a detergent solution, dried thoroughly and wiped out using a hypochlorite, e.g. 1 Sanichlor tablet per litre. Bowls should be stored inverted without being stacked.
- All clinical waste should be tied up and disposed of in the appropriate yellow bags in accordance with the local infection control and disposal of clinical waste policy.
- Equipment belonging to clinics, such as mops, pans and brushes, buckets, aprons and towels should be colour coded or marked to ensure that they remain within the one clinical area.
- Spillage of blood should be washed away with hypochlorite 10 000 ppm in accordance with the local infection control policy.
- Urine and vomit should be removed with detergent and water only before the area is cleaned with hypochlorite 10 000 ppm; this reduces the risk of releasing toxic gas.
- A spillage mop and bucket should be kept in each clinical area.
- Sharps disposal should be in accordance with the local policy. Needles should not be resheathed. Needle stick injuries should be reported in accordance with local policy.
- All accidents should be reported to the Occupational Health Department.

CELLULITIS

This is an inflammation, usually of subcutaneous connective tissue, which produces an area of oedema, heat and a typical brownish appearance. It is commonly found in the lower limbs and results from the penetration of infection into the tissues (Table 7.2). Microorganisms commonly found in association with leg ulcers are listed in Table 7.3.

ISCHAEMIC ULCERATION

In the presence of ischaemic ulceration as seen in Figure 2.9 (C), ulcers will need to be managed using conventional wound care products *and no compression bandages*. Treatment of the underlying cause—for example, bypass arterial reconstruction surgery, if appropriate—will be required to ensure adequate perfusion of oxygen and of nutrients essential to wound healing.

Pain will need to be managed sensitively. Keeping the limbs in the dependent position may enhance perfusion.

Table 7.2 Types of wound infection

Type	Underlying causes	Presentation
Local	Inappropriate wound management	Inflammation at the wound site
		Offensive odour
	Presence of dead tissue	Increased discharge which may be purulent or bloodstained
	Poor immunity	Pain, especially when touched
		Granulation tissue friable and bleeds when lightly touched
Cellulitis	Spread of organisms and toxins into adjacent tissues	Skin is thickened, brownish hue, tender when under pressure
		Pain
		Lymph nodes may be enlarged and tender
	Possible raised blood sugar	Localized increase in skin temperature
		Positive blood culture during septicaemic phase
	Reduced immune response	Rigor
		Ongoing low-grade pyrexia
	Pre-existing oedema	

Table 7.3 Classification of bacteria

Microorganism	Shape	Gram stain	Common organisms
Aerobes	Rods	−ve	Intestinal bacilli — coliforms, e.g. *Escherichia coli*, *Proteus*, *Pseudomonas*
	Cocci	+ve	*Streptococcus pyogenes*, *Staphylococcus aureus*
Anaerobes (unable to utilize free oxygen)	Rods	−ve	*Clostridium welchii* (gas gangrene)
	Rods	−ve	*Bacteroides*

VENOUS ULCERATION AND COMPRESSION BANDAGING

To ensure effective healing, the underlying venous incompetence will need to be corrected. This can be achieved through compression, elevation and exercise.

Rationale for compression in venous ulceration

The advantage of compression is that it:

• reduces backflow from the deep system to the superficial system, which may put pressure on the valves and cause long-term damage (see Fig. 2.6, which shows how incompetent valves lead to venous reflux)

- aids venous return by increasing the velocity of blood flow in the deep veins
- eliminates oedema by reducing the pressure difference between the capillaries and the tissues (Moffatt & Morison 1995).

Interpretation of ABPI results

The ABPI is only a tool *to be used as part of a full assessment* when one is considering the management of leg ulcers by means of compression bandaging. An ankle brachial pressure index of between 0.8 and 1.2 is a safe range in the absence of small vessel disease.

> Compression should only be applied where there is sufficient perfusion to support this:
>
> - ABPI = 0.9–1.2
> - No evidence of small vessel disease
> - No contraindications, e.g. CCF; vasculitis.

> ABPI
>
> - 1.0 = 100% blood flow
> - 0.9–1.2 = normal range
> - < 0.8 indicates ischaemia
> - > 1.2 suggests falsely elevated pressure
> - Beware of calcification of vessels or inflammation.

- *An ABPI of > 1.2* or circumstances where it is impossible to occlude the systolic signal is indicative of calcification of vessels and may reflect a false reading. It is advisable not to use compression bandaging in the presence of diabetic disease except under the supervision of a vascular consultant.
- *0.9–1.2 = normal range.* Full compression is safe in the absence of other medical contraindications, such as calcification of vessels, severe congestive cardiac failure (CCF), microvessel disease, vasculitis (e.g. rheumatoid arthritis or other collagen disorders).
- *0.9–0.8 = 10–20% reduced blood flow.* Only *consider* using 23 mmHg compression at the ankle after consultation with a vascular consultant and under close supervision.
- *0.8–0.7 = 20–30% reduced blood flow.* Only *consider* using 17 mmHg compression at the ankle after consultation with a vascular consultant and under close supervision.

In the presence of diabetes, rheumatoid arthritis, collagen disorders, or previous CVA or TIA, only apply compression under close medical supervision.

Criteria for layered compression bandaging for venous ulceration

The resting ankle brachial pressure index must be within the normal range. *Compression bandaging should only be applied for the management of venous ulcers when there is no evidence of ischaemia or small vessel disease.*

The ABPI should be checked at 3-monthly intervals.

Effect on oedema

In Chapter 2 consideration was given to three theories which account for poor diffusion between the capillary beds and tissues and the effects of venous incompetence, both of which result in oedema. Stemmer theoretically demonstrated that application of a bandage giving 40 mmHg support will restore the fluid balance to normal (Nelson 1995). The concept of Laplace's Law can be applied to pressure bandages, that is: pressure is proportional to the tension in a bandage × the number of layers, divided by the width of the bandage × the circumference of the limb (originally the radius of the limb). It follows that, if the circumference is smaller, the pressure will be larger, and vice versa.

Bandage pressure is inversely proportional to its width; therefore a narrow bandage will exert a higher pressure than a wider one. 10 cm bandages are normally advocated in layered bandage systems.

Bandage tension is also determined by:

- the degree of stretch
- the number of elastic fibres
- how frequently the bandage has been washed
- how long the bandage has been in place.

■ BOX 7.2

Laplace's Law

Sub-bandage pressure is expressed as:

Pressure is proportional to:

$$\frac{\text{number of layers of bandage} \times \text{the bandage tension}}{\text{circumference of the limb} \times \text{the width of the bandage}}$$

Types of compression bandages

- *Short-stretch:* 20–40 mmHg pressure. The differential in pressure depends on the mobility of the patient as the calf muscle is squeezed against an unforgiving weave.
- *Long-stretch Elastomer bandages*, e.g. Tensopress, Setopress, Plastex 23. These all give a sub-bandage pressure of 30–40 mmHg.
- *Layered compression.* The functions of each layer are:
  — *1st layer: cotton wool.* Protects skin and absorbs moisture. One should ensure that there is sufficient padding from this layer to protect skin along the bony prominences from extreme pressure;
  — *2nd layer:* grade 2 support bandage; *crepe layer.* Provides a smooth surface against which to apply compression;
  — *3rd layer: 3a compression 17 mmHg light elastic bandage.* Reduces venous hypertension by aiding venous return;
  — *4th layer: 3b compression cohesive bandage giving 23 mmHg pressure.* Increases level of compression and *sustains* pressure (Fig. 7.2).

Fig. 7.2 Layers or bandages that may be used in applying 40 mmHg compression at the ankle when the ankle circumference is 18–25 cm. (Reproduced with kind permission from Smith & Nephew.)

Fig. 7.2 (A) Cotton wool layer.

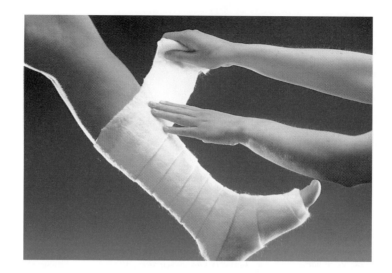

Fig. 7.2 (B) Crepe layer.

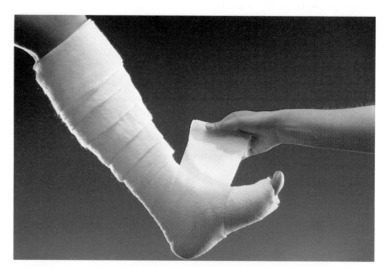

Fig. 7.2 (C) 17 mmHg elastic bandage.

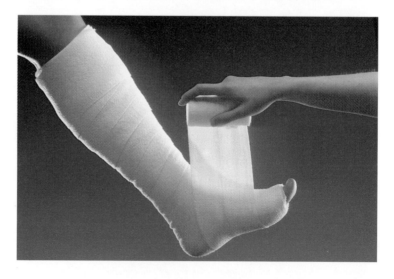

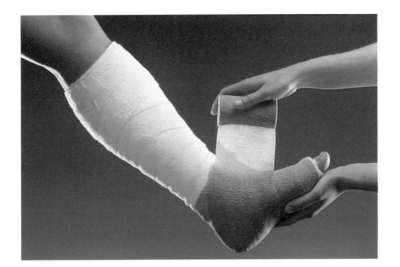

Fig. 7.2 (D) 23 mmHg elastic bandage.

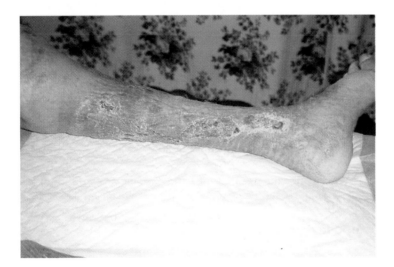

Fig. 7.2 (E) Healed ulcer.

Application of a four-layer bandage (Figs 7.3, 7.4)

• Prior to applying compression bandages, the ankle circumference should be measured if it is the first application and the appropriate bandages selected for treatment. Review of the ankle circumference should be evaluated as the oedema is reduced. ABPI should also be reassessed at regular intervals.

• Informed consent should be obtained and documented. If the patient understands the logistics of compression therapy and the bandage system chosen, compliance may be enhanced. It is important to ensure that the patient has suitable footwear to accommodate the bandages.

• An emollient should be applied to the skin, as prescribed. Those free of lanolin, perfume and parabenz are most appropriate.

• The primary dressing should be applied according to the status of the wound bed.

• The foot should be kept at a 90° angle during application of the bandage.

Wool layer

• Don't stretch this during application. Simply lay onto the leg in a spiral starting from the base of the toes.

• Take around the ankle and slightly catch in the heel.

• Bring the bandage under the base of the foot.

• Spiral up the leg, using a 50% overlap to just below the knee.

• Cotton wool layers can be double wrapped to give extra protection along the tibial crest, or a long strip may be extended along the length of the tibia. If the ankle circumference is less than 18 cm, a double layer will automatically need to be applied.

• Padding may be needed behind hollow ankle bones or to protect prominent joints.

• Where champagne legs present, extra padding around the ankle should help to bring the shape of the leg to allow compression to be applied easily.

Crepe layer

• Apply firmly as all tension will be lost after 20 minutes and this bandage is vacuum-packed.

• Take around the foot and spiral up the leg as above.

• Stop short of the cotton wool below the knee.

Elastomer layer

• Anchor as above then proceed up the leg using a figure-of-eight.

• Stop short of the cotton wool below the knee.

• Tension should be at 50% stretch with 50% overlap.

Cohesive layer

• Anchor as for all layers.

• Spiral up the leg at 50% stretch and 50% overlay.

• Stop short of the cotton wool layer.

• Compressive layers should *never* be double wrapped.

• Try not to add in bandages. If this is really necessary only start the new bandage at the edge of the original bandage. Bandages are made in longer lengths.

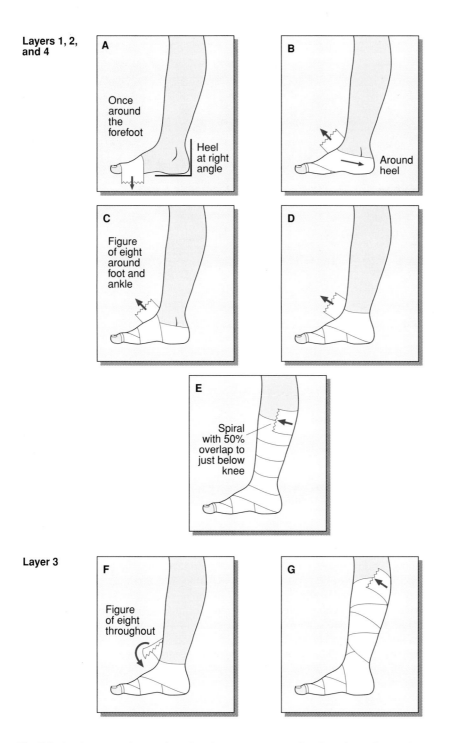

Fig. 7.3 Application technique for a four-layer compression bandage. Layer 3 is similar to layers 1, 2 and 4 but the Figure-of-eight pattern continues up the leg.

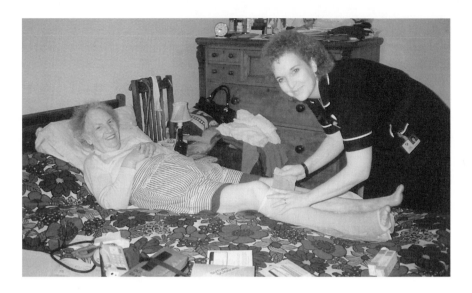

Fig. 7.4 Completed application of a compression bandage by a district nurse. The Charing Cross four-layered system for treatment of a venous leg ulcer has been used.

- Placing two fingers under the bandage where it crosses the Achilles' tendon will help to prevent pressure necrosis.
- Where four-layer bandaging cannot be resourced because of prescribing restrictions, a three-layer system using a cotton wool bandage, crepe and a single 40 mmHg compression bandage may suffice. To support this the ABPI must be between 0.8 and 1.2.

Figure 7.2 (E) shows how effective such a bandage can be: a 13-year-old ulcer was healed within 3 months by the use of a layered compression system.

The advantages of a layered compression system

'A venous ulcer will fail or be slow to heal without the application of *sustained* graduated compression which can only be applied by using elastic bandages' (Moffatt & Morison 1995). They also report that in 1969 Stemmer showed theoretically that graduated compression with an ankle pressure of 40 mmHg would improve effective venous return, while Blair et al (1987) demonstrated that the four-layer system was able to achieve 42 mmHg at the ankle and heal 75% of all venous leg ulcers in 12 weeks.

Comparison of high- and low-pressure compression bandages in healing chronic leg ulcers demonstrated that the four-layer method healed over 70% of chronic venous ulcers which had previously failed to heal with the use of Elastoplast bandages over a period of 2 years. These now healed within 6 weeks (McCullum 1996 & Blair 1988). Four-layer bandaging can maintain graduated sub-bandage pressure ranging from 40 mm at the ankle to 17 mm below the knee for a week, owing to the presence of the cohesive component.

Four-layer bandaging showed a significantly higher rate of healing when compared to high compression and paste and crepe.

By using multiple layers of bandages at differing pressures, one obtains an increased safety margin, as pressure is diversified through these layers. This reduces the effect of extra pressure caused by overstretching one single layer.

The layering of compression bandaging ensures versatility. The level of compression can be tailored to meet the individual needs of patients as inferred from their past medical history, ankle brachial pressure index and ankle circumference. This will lead to improved patient compliance.

Moffatt's recommendations for levels of compression when the ankle brachial pressure is within the normal range are given in Table 7.4.

The following points should also be noted:

- It is essential that the ankle circumference be measured on the first assessment and 1 week later when the oedema has reduced.

| Ankle circumference and ABPI should be regularly reviewed. |

- *After* application the patient should be warned to inspect the toes repeatedly for discoloration and note excessive pins and needles, loss of sensation or unusual levels of pain in the calf or foot. Should any of these signs become excessive, the bandage should be cut off. Leave a contact telephone number.

- *The status of perfusion in the patient's leg and foot should be checked* for 24 hours after the first application.

- When the ulcer or venous eczema has healed, the bandage should be left in place for 1–2 weeks to enhance the tensile strength of newly formed collagen.

One should ensure that the patient is fitted for compression hosiery before the ulcer has healed. The use of a stocking applicator may be of assistance in permitting the easy application of hosiery and therefore improving compliance. Stockings should be renewed every 3 months, when the patient is reviewed.

| Compression hosiery is essential in preventing recurrence of venous leg ulcers. |

The use of compression hosiery may also help to reduce lipodermatosclerosis reforming. For cosmetic purposes, one may wish to promote fibrinolysis further by the use of a fibrinolytic agent such as stanozolol.

The patient should be educated with regard to ways of preventing recurrent leg ulceration and lipodermatosclerosis—such as sitting with legs elevated, not standing for long periods, pursuing a healthy lifestyle and adhering to a regime of leg exercises.

Table 7.4 Recommendations for compression levels (after Moffatt & Morison 1995)

Ankle circum- ference	Inner layer	Second layer	Third layer	Top layer
< 18 cm	2 or more wool layers	1 crepe	1 17 mmHg elastic bandage	1 23 mmHg cohesive bandage
18–25 cm	1 wool layer	1 crepe	1 17 mmHg elastic bandage	1 23 mmHg cohesive bandage
25–30 cm	1 wool layer	1 crepe	1 40 mmHg elastic bandage	1 23 mmHg cohesive bandage
> 30 cm	1 wool layer	1 17 mmHg elastic bandage	1 40 mmHg elastic bandage	1 23 mmHg cohesive bandage

MIXED AETIOLOGY ULCERS

Paste bandages and light compression still have a role to play in promoting healing and protecting the surrounding skin. For centuries, medicated zinc bandages have been found to have a soothing and beneficial effect on leg ulcers. Zinc may increase cell mitosis and proliferation, strengthen collagen cross-bonding, reduce free radical activity and inhibit bacterial growth, so influencing wound healing (Anderson 1995).

The efficacy of oral zinc in wound healing is unclear. If the patient has a low plasma zinc, receiving oral zinc does improve healing, but this is not the case if the zinc level is normal.

Topical zinc application is less likely to have adverse effects on the patient, such as gastric upset and interactions with copper and iron. Zinc inhibits copper metabolism and iron therapy interferes with zinc. If zinc and castor oil cream is used to protect surrounding tissues, care needs to be taken to ensure that the tissues are carefully washed; otherwise an unhealthy build-up of cream may occur. Turner suggests that:

> more needs to be understood about the role of topical zinc in wound healing, absorption rates and the amount of zinc required if it is to enhance healing. Zinc-paste bandages with an amended formula, reducing the incidence of reaction, may offer nurses a valuable tool within the parameters of the ideal dressing. (Turner 1985)

Empirically, zinc bandages are more effective than oral zinc, but this may be due to poor delivery of zinc via diseased vessels, the direct effect of the bandage or the antibacterial effect of zinc oxide.

MANAGEMENT OF UNDERLYING MEDICAL CONDITIONS AND RISK FACTORS

If it is to promote healing, nursing management will need to address any underlying medical conditions by providing the required nursing intervention. For example, patients presenting with diabetes will need to attend to control of blood sugar levels and to ensure that suitable footwear is worn. Those with an inflammatory disease such as rheumatoid arthritis may require anti-inflammatory medication.

Attention will need to be given to the patient's medication to identify any drugs that may have an adverse effect on wound healing. Cytotoxics and steroids will both alter the tensile strength of tissues. Beta-blockers will cause vasoconstriction, reducing the perfusion of oxygen and nutrients to wounds. It has been demonstrated that histamine H_2 receptor antagonists, and other agents that significantly reduce gastric acid production, may reduce the ability of the body to absorb vitamin B_{12}, resulting in a macrocytic anaemia and consequent leg ulceration. A presentation of ulceration coexisting with loss of memory, dementia or psychosis should alert the practitioner to the need to review medication (Jorden et al 1996).

Addressing lifestyle issues, such as smoking, obesity, psychosocial issues, stress and lack of exercise will all help to reduce the risk of ulceration.

ALTERNATIVE THERAPIES IN THE PROMOTION OF WOUND HEALING

Simple leg elevation at 45°

Leg elevation is beneficial when leg ulceration is extensive and heavily exudating, so requiring daily dressings. Poor patient compliance may be improved by admission to hospital, but where possible it is preferable to support patients in their own homes.

Intermittent pneumatic compression (IPC) (Fig. 6.2)

This is effective in reducing oedema and enabling essential oxygen to reach the tissues, so promoting wound healing. It has been widely used in the prevention of deep vein thrombosis and in aiding lymphatic drainage; it is virtually the only effective treatment for chronic lymphoedema.

For reduction of oedema, it has been demonstrated that the most acceptable levels of intermittent compression in a non-ischaemic patient are 15 seconds inflation at a maximum of 400 mmHg pressure, followed by 12 seconds deflation (Grieveson et al 1994).

Hyperbaric oxygen therapy

The aim of treatment is to improve healing by intermittently increasing the oxygenation of plasma, hence elevating oxygen tissue tension at the wound site. It is thought that perfusion of tissues with such plasma may be sufficient to ensure tissue viability in the absence of adequate haemoglobin levels of oxygen.

Wound healing may be impaired, particularly in the presence of ischaemia, chronic venous incompetence, infection, diabetes mellitus, radiotherapy and chemotherapy. Wound healing demands a higher oxygen tension. The administration of hyperbaric oxygen increases tissue oxygen tension, so promoting angiogenesis, enhanced collagen formation, fibroblast replication and improved leucocyte function (Hammarlund & Sundberg 1993). This leads to an increased resistance to bacteria, particularly anaerobes.

The vasoconstrictive action of oxygen does not seem to interfere with the delivery of oxygen to the tissues, but rather helps to reduce localized oedema by closing the pores along the length of the microcirculatory vessels.

In normal respiration at atmospheric pressure, the patient's usual oxygen-carrying capacity is 0.3 ml of oxygen per 100 ml of plasma. Under hyperbaric conditions the patient breathes 100% oxygen under pressure three times greater than normal atmospheric pressure. The oxygen-carrying capacity of the plasma increases to 6.5 ml of oxygen per 100 ml of plasma—over 20 times greater than normal.

Impressive results in wound healing have been demonstrated in recent case studies managed at the Tissue Repair Research Unit at Guy's and St Thomas' Medical School in London (Miller 1995).

Hyperbaric oxygen therapy may be delivered from a large chamber.

Currently, work is under way to assess the effectiveness of topical delivery using specially manufactured bags that will stand high pressures. The results of clinical trials are so far variable, but on balance seem promising.

Low-level laser therapy (LLLT)

LLLT involves the application of light over injuries or wounds to stimulate healing. It effectively induces pain relief, resolves inflammation, increases the speed of healing and enhances the quality and tensile strength of new tissues. LLLT also boosts the immune system, so aiding the resolution of infection (Fig. 7.5).

These effects are achieved by 3B lasers which emit sufficient radiation to stimulate an increase in mast cell, macrophage and fibroblast populations and a speeding up of the healing process.

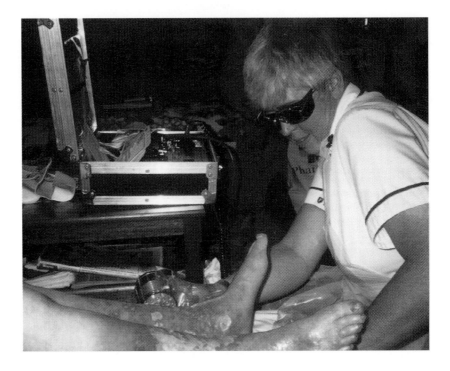

Fig. 7.5 The application of low-level laser therapy to aid wound healing and boost the immune system.

REFERENCES

Anderson I 1995 Zinc as an aid to healing. Nursing Times 91(30) Wound Care Supplement
Blair S et al 1987 Comparison of high and low pressure compression bandages in healing chronic venous leg ulcers. Swiss Medicine 10(44): 111–112
Blair S et al 1987 What compression heals chronic venous ulcer? British Jn Surg 74: 529–535
Blair S 1988 Do dressings influence the healing of chronic venous ulcers? Phlebology 3: 129–134
Grieveson S, Rithalia S, Gonsalkarale P 1994 Most effective settings of intermittent pneumatic compression pump for reduction of oedema. (Unpublished)
Hammarlund C, Sundberg T 1993 Hyperbaric oxygen reduced size of chronic leg ulcers: randomised double blind study. 93(4): 829–833
Jorden J et al 1996 Bionursing: side effects of ulcer treatment. Nursing Standard 10(16): 30–32
McCullum C N 1993 An audit system to evaluate venous ulcer care in the community. (Stockport Audit Department of Surgery.) Unpublished work.
McCullum C N 1996 Audit system to achieve venous ulcer care in the the community. British Medical Journal 132: 1648–1651
Miller M 1994 The ideal healing environment. Nursing Times 90(45): 62–68
Miller M 1995 Use of oxygen therapy. Nursing Times 91(30): 64–68
Moffatt C, Morison M 1995 A colour guide to the assessment and management of leg ulcers, 2nd edn. Mosby, Edinburgh
Morgan D 1994 Formulary of wound care products. Euromed Communications. Hademere, Surrey
Nelson A 1995 Compression bandaging for venous leg ulcers. Journal of Tissue Viability 5(2): 57–62
Turner T D 1985 Which dressing and why? In: Westby S (ed) Wound care. Heinemann, London
Wilson J 1995 Infection control in clinical practice. Baillière Tindall, London

FURTHER READING

Bird A D, Telfer A B M 1965 The effect of hyperbaric oxygen on limb circulation. Lancet 1: 355

Blair S et al 1988 Do dressings influence the healing of venous leg ulcers. Journal of Phlebology 3: 129–134

Cameron J 1991 The consequences of incorrect Doppler ultrasound in differential diagnosis of venous and arterial lower limb pathologies. Nursing Standard 40: 25–27

Cullum N 1994a Leg ulcer management, a research based guide. Scutari, London

Cullum N 1994b Nursing management of leg ulcers in the community. Liverpool University Press, Liverpool

Cullum N, Roe B 1995 Leg ulcer management. Scutari, London

Dale J J et al 1983 How efficient is a compression bandage? Nursing Times 79: 49–51

Dale J J et al 1985 Chronic ulcers of the leg: a study of prevalence in a Scottish community. Health Bulletin 41: 310–314

Dimond B 1990 Legal aspects of nursing. Prentice-Hall, Englewood Cliffs, NJ

Ertl P 1991 Incidence and aetiology of leg ulcers. Professional Nurse 3: 190–194

Ertl P 1992 Looking beyond the ulcer itself. Assessment of leg ulcers. Professional Nurse 4: 258–262

Ertl P 1993 The multi benefits of accurate assessment. Professional Nurse 912: 139–144

Franks P, Moffatt C, Connolly M et al 1995 Factors associated with healing leg ulceration with high compression. Age and Aging 24: 407–410

Franks P, Oldroyd M I, Dickson D et al 1995 Risk factors for leg ulcer recurrence: a randomised trial of two types of compression stocking. Age and Aging 24: 490–494

Griffiths-Jones A 1995 Methicillin resistant *Staphylococcus aureus* in wound care. Journal of Wound Care 4(10): 481–483

Heng M C Y 1983 Hyperbaric oxygen therapy for a foot ulcer in a patient with polyarteris nodosa. Australian Journal of Dermatology 120: 640–645

Jeffcoate W, MacFarlane R 1995 The diabetic foot: an illustrated guide to management. Chapman & Hall Medical, London

Lambourne L 1993 Bedfordshire audit. Research Update, October

Lees T A, Lambert D 1992 Prevalence of lower limb ulceration in an urban health district. British Journal of Surgery 79: 1032–1034

Logan J et al 1993 A comparison of sub-bandage pressures produced by experienced and inexperienced bandagers. Journal of Wound Care 1(3)

McIntosh J B 1979 Decision making on the district. Nursing Times 75(29): 77–80

Moffatt C 1993 Community clinics for venous leg ulcers – an impact on healing. British Medical Journal 305: 1389–1392

Moffat C 1995 Graduated compression hosiery for venous ulceration. Journal of Wound Care 4(10): 459–462

Nelson A 1995 Compression bandaging for venous leg ulcers. Journal of Tissue Viability 15(2): 57–61

Roe B et al 1993 Prevention and monitoring of chronic leg ulcers in the community. Journal of Clinical Nursing 5: 299–306

Thomas S 1995 Wound management and dressings. Pharmacology Press, London

Williams A 1994 The Hope removal walking cast: a method of treatment for diabetic/neuropathic ulceration. Practical Diabetes 11(1): 20–23

Wilson J 1995 Infection control in clinical practice. Baillière Tindall, London

CHAPTER 8

Caring for the patient with chronic ischaemia

This chapter discusses the patient with *chronic ischaemia*, which may be caused by long-term arterial occlusion due to vasospastic disorders, Buerger's disease, thromboembolus, inflammation, diabetic disease, atherosclerotic disease and calcification of vessels. Chronic ischaemia may produce minimal symptoms in the early stages, or may present with pain, ulceration or gangrene. It has been determined that atherosclerosis is a significant cause of morbidity and mortality in peripheral arterial disease (Fowkes et al 1992).

The major cause of chronic ischaemia is atherosclerosis.

Patients may be maintained over many years before they present with severe claudication or critical ischaemia, as discussed in Chapter 9.

The lack of diffusion from the peripheral circulation to the tissues of nutrients and oxygen results in cell death. Damage to the endothelial lining of the vessels can arise as a result of activated neutrophils, chemical mediators and free radicals entering the systemic circulation following a mild period of ischaemia, such as may have occurred in intermittent claudication (Green & Shearman 1994).

Leng's work suggests that, in 8% of cases, the presence of major arterial disease may be asymptomatic, and post-mortem studies have found significant stenotic disease in as many as 15% of men and 5% of women (Leng & Fowkes 1993).

As peripheral vascular disease is often associated with a certain lifestyle, it is theoretically possible to improve the situation by reducing risk factors such as smoking, inadequate exercise levels and hypertension. An incorrect diet may lead to obesity or may contain a high level of saturated fat predisposing to atheroma, or may provoke poorly controlled diabetes, leading to hyperglycaemia. Factors which cannot be changed are gender, hereditary abnormalities and age.

Where a chronic situation is exacerbated by an acute episode, or where there is a single acute episode resulting in critical ischaemia as discussed in Chapter 9, vascular reconstructive surgery may be indicated. Should a chronic situation become so severe that the patient no longer enjoys a reasonable quality of life, further intervention may also be considered.

Peripheral vascular disease rarely presents in isolation. Coronary heart disease and cerebrovascular accidents are often found to coexist—a fact that must be taken into account in relation to the needs and management of this patient group.

MANAGEMENT OF PATIENTS WITH SMALL VESSEL DISEASE

Vasospastic disorders

Acrocyanosis and livedo reticularis may present with constant ischaemic changes in the upper extremities but ulceration is not common. Acrocyanosis and livedo reticularis are difficult to distinguish from Raynaud's phenomenon, except that it presents with continuous rather than intermittent symptoms and signs; again, skin ulceration does not usually present. However, when Raynaud's phenomenon occurs with collagen and vascular disorders, ulceration is not uncommon. As treatment of the two conditions is not dissimilar, differential diagnosis is not critical.

Raynaud's phenomenon and Raynaud's disease may present with a history of numbness or extreme pain in the fingertips. The skin of the fingers may systematically pass through colour changes ranging from pale to cyanosed to red when the ambient temperature varies or when the patient is experiencing anxiety. The hands may feel cold. Nails may be fissured and fingertips may be tapered—a consequence of scarring from previous ulceration. In the later stages, ulcers or gangrene may be apparent on the fingertips. Axillary, brachial and radial pulses are not usually affected by vasospastic disorders.

Obtaining a full medical history will help to identify Raynaud's phenomenon. This is associated with many aetiologies, which can be divided into the following groups:

- systemic diseases and conditions such as cold haemagglutination or cryoglobulinaemia, myxoedema and ergotism
- *occupational trauma* induced by vibration, and activities which require tapping of the digits, e.g. typing and piano playing
- *compression of the nerves*, as found in carpal tunnel syndrome and thoracic outlet syndrome
- *arterial occlusive disease* associated with atherosclerosis
- vasculitis associated with diabetes, rheumatoid arthritis, autoimmune disorders and Buerger's disease.

Differential diagnosis in small vessel disease

This will be determined from the presenting clinical signs and history. Investigations which may be undertaken are:

- digital temperature recovery time
- Doppler flow velocity detection
- arteriography
- digital plethysmography
- blood screening for platelets to eliminate any association with thrombocytosis
- ESR to help determine whether there is systemic disease
- levels of cryoglobulins, macrogobulins and cold agglutinins (these are proteins that may coagulate in cold temperatures, so occluding the vascular system)
- immunological factors, including RA latex and antinuclear factor (ANF), which is indicative of lupus erythematosus.
- a skin biopsy, which may help to provide an objective diagnosis.

Conservative management of patients with small vessel disease and vasospastic disorders

- Wherever possible the underlying cause should be addressed, as well as the presenting clinical factors.
- Protection of the limb from hazards within the environment needs to be assured.
- The patient should be encouraged to keep warm by the use of thermal clothing, and can be referred to the appliance officer for electric warming gloves.
- Information relating to self-help groups—e.g. the Raynaud's Association Trust—may help patients to feel less isolated (see Appendix 1).
- Tobacco should always be avoided. The patient should be given information about the effects of tobacco and cold on the circulation in order to promote compliance.
- Calcium-blocking agents such as nifedipine and alpha-adrenergic blocking

drugs such as thymoxamine may help to reduce vasoconstriction. As an alternative, guanethidine may be combined with prazosin in a bid to reduce side-effects from medication. Drug therapy is contraindicated if the patient experiences side-effects such as nausea, dizziness, palpitation, headache, flushing or oedema.

• For patients in whom vasospasticity is induced by stress and anxiety, thermal biofeedback training may be supportive. This has proved successful in 80–90% of people with Raynaud's phenomenon.

Intravenous prostaglandin therapy

This may promote vasodilatation and a reduction in platelet aggregation, so reducing coagulation. It may also be used as an adjunct to sympathectomy, which is discussed later in this chapter, or in conjunction with reconstruction surgery, either pre-operatively or postoperatively, until perfusion has picked up.

Prostaglandins have a half-life of around 30 minutes; therefore, if the patient's blood pressure drops to below 100/50, the infusion should be immediately stopped for at least 30 minutes before the therapy is continued.

During this procedure the patient should be closely monitored for bradycardia associated with hypotension, increased pallor, nausea, abdominal pain and sweating. As the heart has become used to working against a high intravascular pressure, a reduction in pressure will excite the heart, resulting in tachycardia and the risk of myocardial infarction.

The benefits of treatment, including the temperature and colour of the skin, should be recorded at regular intervals. Side-effects include dryness of the mouth, raised serum glucose, flushing, headache, nausea, vomiting, gastric upsets, chest pain and tightness and pain over the infusion site.

Dosage is normally weight-related, and therefore the patient will need to be weighed. The maximum benefit of treatment will be gained within 5 days, after which the effect will plateau out. It is not advisable to continue treatment for longer than 7 days. Prostaglandin therapy will usually go on enhancing perfusion for 3 to 6 months after administration.

Relative contraindications are specifically confined to pregnancy and lactation, at the discretion of medical staff. To date, however, there is little available evidence regarding the effect of the therapy on the unborn child and on lactation.

Sympathectomy

This procedure is undertaken where there is oversensitivity of the sympathetic system, resulting in vasospasm, since it denervates the sympathetic nervous system which would normally control vascular tone. It is useful in alleviating vasoconstriction, and so permitting enhanced perfusion that will result in a reduction in pain, ulceration and ischaemia. Sympathectomy is used to treat vasospastic leg ulceration. Other indications are hyperhidrosis and post-traumatic pain.

The sympathetic chain stimulates vascular tone and sweat glands. Under normal conditions, the sympathetic nervous system causes only the amount of vasoconstriction necessary to keep the extremities warm, dry and comfortable without supplying the parts with too much blood. As environmental conditions change, sympathetic stimuli alternately vasoconstrict or vasodilate the peripheral vessels in accordance with the subtle variations in the body's need for heat transfer and tissue maintenance (LeMaitre & Finnegan 1980).

Sympathectomy will only reduce vasoconstriction in the small vessels of the skin, so that they become warm and pink. It does not increase muscle blood flow or benefit claudication in any way. It is therefore probably best suited to those presenting with thromboangiitis obliterans or vasospasm. Where major vessels are occluded, sympathectomy has an uncertain role (Forrest et al 1985). The success of

---

Conservative management of small vessel disease:

• identify cause and treat cause if possible
• relieve anxiety
• relieve pain
• promote sleep during the night
• possibly elevate head of bed to aid arterial supply
• protect limb
• promote exercise to develop collateral blood supply
• keep warm
• address lifestyle issues
• stop patient smoking
• help patient to avoid stress
• give medication
• encourage participation in self-help groups.

Sympathectomy promotes:

• reduction in vasospasm
• reduction in vasoconstriction of small vessels
• elimination of hyperhidrosis
• improvement for up to 6 months

It does not increase muscle blood flow in the presence of intermittent claudication.

sympathectomy can be short-lived, and it is not uncommon for symptoms to present anew after 3–6 months.

Where the ABPI is greater than 0.35 and patients are presenting with primary Raynaud's disease without coexisting systemic, autoimmune or collagen disorders, sympathectomy may be indicated to reduce vasoconstriction in either the upper or lower extremity, especially if the patient has ulcerated limbs. The success of this procedure is greater for vasospasm affecting the lower limbs, but the reason for this is not known.

When sympathetic denervation is required to relieve symptoms in the upper limbs, sympathectomy may be achieved by open or laparoscopic cervical surgery. Access to the cervical ganglion during laparoscopic surgery is through the axilla. The lung is deflated by the anaesthetist and the pleural space filled with carbon dioxide. The appropriate ganglia are identified and cauterized, and the carbon dioxide is sucked out of the lung, thereby reflating it. The procedure is repeated on the other side.

For vasospastic disorders of the lower limbs, a lumbar neurolytic block may be considered; this denervates the motor pathways that are producing vasoconstriction and the sensory pathways that are normally responsible for vascular pain conduction. To access the lumbar ganglia, the surgeon inserts a needle under radiographic control at around L3/L4; when the ganglia have been located in the retroperitoneal space, the nerves are destroyed with phenol.

Post-surgical sympathectomy

Following cervical sympathectomy the patient may be nursed with a chest drain, as it is necessary to collapse the lung during this procedure.

- Limbs need to be checked for the presence of pulses.
- Limbs should be observed for colour and skin temperature.

Buerger's disease:

- mainly found in males under 40
- smoking cessation is rarely possible
- thrombophlebitis in medium and small vessels
- followed by disease of major vessels and collaterals
- leads to ulceration and gangrene.

MANAGEMENT OF THE PATIENT WITH BUERGER'S DISEASE (THROMBOANGIITIS OBLITERANS)

Sadly, Buerger's disease is a degenerative condition found mainly in men, and occasionally women, under the age of 40 who are unable to stop smoking. Thrombophlebitis in the medium-sized veins and arteries is induced by cigarette smoking, and eventually the disease process affects the major vessels and collaterals as thrombus is formed. This results in ulceration of the limbs and gangrene.

Investigations may include:

- blood screening for full blood count and ESR
- angiography.

Nursing management

The patient and his relatives will require a substantial amount of psychological and emotional support. This disease affects people who would otherwise be in the prime of their lives. While they understand fully the effects of smoking on their health, they experience great difficulty in stopping, in spite of the evidence of devastating physical changes. The family may well not understand why, given the consequences of continued smoking, the patient is unable to stop. Every support in smoking cessation should be given to patients and their families.

The following points are important in managing such patients:

- Assessment and protection of pressure areas and limbs are essential.
- A bed cradle may help to relieve pressure from bed linen.
- Elevation of the head of the bed will keep the lower limbs dependent, thereby aiding perfusion.
- A nutritious diet will assist the body's repair process.

Referral to social services for advice regarding financial benefits, mobility allowance, rehousing or placement in a nursing home, home care and meals on wheels is often necessary. Should the patient lose a limb or become wheelchair-bound, alterations to the home may be necessary. Job retraining can improve the quality of life and help the patient to secure an income and actualization. The enhanced self-esteem that this generates often reinforces patients' efforts to stop smoking.

It is often necessary to refer these patients to the physiotherapist and occupational therapist, as they need help with mobility and with the provision of home aids.

Pain should be carefully monitored and appropriate analgesia administered. Aspirin may also be administered to effect a reduction in the viscosity of the blood, as discussed in Chapter 13.

Any ulcerated areas will need to be managed, as discussed in Chapter 6. Should the patient eventually require amputation, the procedure outlined in Chapter 10 should be followed.

CARING FOR THE PATIENT WITH CLAUDICATION

> Claudication = pain associated with walking:
>
> - mild disease: claudication at over 100 m
> - moderated disease: claudication at 100 m
> - severe disease: less than 100 metres with a post-exercise ankle pressure of < 50 mmHg

'Claudication' comes from the Latin *'claudus'*, meaning 'lame', somewhat dubiously attributed to the Emperor Claudius who walked with a limp. Hence today we have the word *claudication* which is defined as pain brought on when walking. It is most frequently experienced in the buttocks, calf or feet, depending on the level of occlusion. The cramp-like pain will be experienced distal to the occlusion.

Patients with chronic ischaemia who are not critical may present in category 1 or 2 as listed below. Category 3 relates to patients with critical ischaemia, as discussed in Chapter 9.

Cascade of pain

Category 1:
Pain associated with levels of intermittent claudication
a. Mild disease: able to walk for 5 minutes at 2 miles per hour on a 12% incline. Ankle pressure after exercise > 50 mmHg or an ABPI of > 0.6.
b. Moderate disease: worse than (a) above, but not as severe as (c) below.
c. Significant disease: cannot complete treadmill test. Ankle pressure after exercise < 50 mmHg.

Category 2: pain at rest
Ankle pressure less than 40 mmHg or an ABPI of < 0.3 with a monophasic Doppler signal. Pain may be experienced during the night when the leg is elevated and the metabolic rate drops.

Category 3: tissue loss in the presence of severe rest pain and nocturnal pain

a. Minor loss: resting ankle pressure < 60 mmHg with monophasic Doppler reading; clinically non-healing ulcer and/or focal gangrene.
b. Major loss of tissues; flat Doppler wave form.

Assessment of the effectiveness of pain control needs to be maintained.

The biggest causative factor of claudication is atherosclerosis of the major vessels of the leg.

Fontaine's classification of ischaemia

Fontaine classified chronic ischaemia of the lower limbs into four grades of symptoms and signs:

1. Asymptomatic.
2. Intermittent claudication.
3. Severe persistent pain at rest caused by arterial disease.
4. Arterial disease, resulting in severe rest pain associated with ulceration and/or gangrene.

Patients may have found that over a period of time the distance they are able to walk on the level before needing to stop and recover from the pain has decreased, and is even less if they are walking on an incline. On Doppler assessment there are normally significantly reduced pressures of less than 0.8 mmHg, depending on the degree of occlusion. The colour of the foot may be pale or cyanosed or it may present with dependent rubor. The extremity of the limb may feel cooler than the remaining part of the limb or the contralateral limb. Claudication may also be associated with degenerative disease of the hip or neurospinal conditions with involvement of the sympathetic nerves.

Rest pain and pain at night may be relieved by hanging the foot down. During sleep the cardiac output is reduced, and this reduction will place extra strain on the tissues supplied by the peripheral vessels.

Conservative management

Reconstructive surgery is reserved for critically ischaemic situations which threaten a limb, or for when the severity of ischaemic pain has become intolerable. In these situations there is much to be gained through surgical intervention.

While bypass reconstructive surgery is effective in 70% of cases, it is not without risks. Therefore, it is important to maintain this patient group for as long as possible by conservative management. Should a graft become occluded by thrombus or infection, the patient may be worse off than when coping with claudication. The success of reconstructive surgery is reduced if an autologous vein graft is not available, as synthetic grafts are not fed by the vasa vasorum. It may not be feasible to regraft, and therefore amputation may be required should complications arise.

The mainstay of conservative treatment is exercise. As early as 1966 Larsen and Lassen proved in a controlled trial that exercise training of claudicants over 1 year produced a 300% increase in walking distance compared with controls. With intense training patients may become symptom-free, despite the fact that there is no change on Doppler measurement or on angiogram. With exercise, walking distance can double in 2 months (Ernst & Matrai 1987). However, in advanced cases of stenosis, where the oxygen demand of the exercising muscles is overwhelming, brisk walking may be unacceptable because the pain is intolerable. In these circumstances, selectively chosen exercises within the limits of the individual can still help to stimulate a collateral blood supply. Care needs to be taken when exercising patients with cardiopulmonary disease and strict protocols need to be adhered to.

Chronic ischaemia = long-term degeneration of arterial perfusion resulting from:

- occlusive disease (atherosclerosis)
- vasospasm
- vasculitis
- aneurysmal disease.

Conservative management for large vessel disease:

- psychological support
- pain relief
- exercise to enhance collateral supply
- elevation of head of bed to enhance blood supply at night, so enhancing sleep
- addressing lifestyle issues—health promotion
- skin care
- nutrition.

The reasons for improvement are only speculative (Ernst 1991):

* haemodynamic: dilatation of collaterals and capillaries with redistribution of flow
* metabolic: changes in mitochondria in the cells leading to improved respiration
* structural: growth of new collaterals and capillaries
* psychological: improved self-image leading to patient stopping smoking, etc.

Conservative management over a course of 6–8 weeks may produce an improvement as the collateral vessels develop. Assessing the patient for 3–6 months will help medical staff to determine his or her long-term management.

Oral vasodilators

Vasodilatory medication is discussed in Chapter 13.

Assessment of the claudicant patient

Objective investigations to determine the cause of the claudication could include treadmill assessment, pre- and post-exercise Doppler ultrasound assessment of the ankle brachial pressure index, and straight X-rays of the hips and spinal column. Treadmill assessment is discussed in Chapter 5.

Conservative management plan

Should it be determined that the cause of claudication is vascular, an appropriate management plan will need to be devised. This may involve a non-invasive programme which addresses lifestyle issues and which includes a structured exercise programme to develop the collateral blood supply. The use of vasodilating drugs can sometimes help. Invasive action in the form of percutaneous balloon angioplasty, reconstruction bypass surgery or the insertion of a stent may be indicated. The proportion of patients with claudication who go on to need an amputation is as low as 5–10% (Hallett et al 1995).

Conservative nursing management of claudicant patients is outlined in Table 8.1. Patients with intermittent claudication will need ongoing assessment of their degree of claudication and of how much it is interfering with their everyday activities. The progress of patients being cared for under a conservative management programme may be mapped on a graph to highlight the benefits gained by following the programme. One can plot, for instance, the distances walked over a set period of time, as well as other targets such as stopping smoking and weight reduction. Patients will feel motivated when they see the positive effects that stopping smoking and regular exercise can have on the peripheral circulation, as demonstrated by a reduction in symptoms.

PERCUTANEOUS TRANSLUMINAL ANGIOPLASTY

In 1964, Dotter and Judkins were the first to describe transluminal percutaneous angioplasty (PTA), but it was only in 1976, when Gruntzig introduced the double lumen balloon catheter, that this technique was accepted as being a suitable treatment to relieve stenosis in all the major peripheral vessels and to achieve recanalization.

The procedure for angioplasty

This procedure involves the insertion of a polyethylene catheter that has an inflatable balloon near the tip; it is passed through the stenosis and expanded to compress the atheromatous plaque against the medial lining of the walls of the vessel. Hence the lumen of the vessel becomes patent again.

Table 8.1 Conservative nursing management of claudicant patients

Problem	Goal	Action
Pain when walking	Patient able to extend the distance walked as the collateral blood flow is enhanced	Reduce risk factors contributing to atherosclerosis, e.g.: — smoking
	Leg muscles adapt to anaerobic metabolism	— hypertension — uncontrolled diabetes — high saturated fats in the diet
	Frequency and length of stops when patient is walking decrease	— high levels of stress — obesity
	Pain is controlled or eliminated	Suggest regular additional exercises of the lower limbs for 30 minutes 3–5 times per week
		Teach patient to rest at the onset of pain, but encourage to continue once the pain has subsided, to ensure that a full exercise programme is maintained
		During poor weather conditions, indoor activities should be encouraged, within the limitations of the individual's capabilities, e.g. walking inside an enclosed area, swimming, using an exercise bicycle, performing lower limb exercises from a given programme
		Give analgesic medication as prescribed
The patient smokes	The patient stops smoking	Educate the patient regarding the effects of nicotine and carbon monoxide
	Vasoconstriction is reduced	Suggest the use of nicotine patches or chewing gum to assist in reducing the craving for cigarettes
	Blood flow and diffusion of nutrients and oxygen to the tissues are increased	
		Give the patient advice about stop smoking groups/clinics
Raised serum lipids	Serum lipids are within normal range	Give the patient information regarding the intake of fat in the diet
	Production of atheroma is retarded	Refer to a dietician if necessary
	Total fat and calorific intake per 24 hours is within the recommended range	Keep alcohol consumption within acceptable limits as excess consumption provokes hypertriglyceridaemia
		Administer lipid lowering drugs as prescribed
		Manage stress
Diabetes mellitus—increased risk of ischaemia, infection and neuropathy, resulting in altered gait and sensation	Diabetes mellitus under control	Refer to the dietician if necessary for advice on diabetic diet
	Reduced risk of infection causing poor healing of minor ischaemic ulcers	Ensure footwear is appropriate and does does not cause undue pressure
	Reduced risk of unrecognized trauma caused by loss of sensation and altered pressure on the feet as a result of neuropathy and altered motor control	Educate the patient regarding foot care

Cont'd

Table 8.1 Conservative nursing management of claudicant patients (cont'd)

Problem	Goal	Action
Patient hypersensitive to cold	No discomfort experienced from the environmental temperature	Encourage the use of warm clothing and bed socks, e.g. thermal
		Discourage the use of hot water bottles and sitting by the fire as this may traumatize the tissues
		Discourage long soaks in the bath as this may soften the skin, allowing entry to microorganisms and promoting ulceration
When patient is supine there is reduced blood flow to the lower limbs	Improved perfusion of tissues and patient comfort	Encourage the patient to keep the legs in a dependent position unless this produces oedema
Poor peripheral circulation requiring oral or intravenous medication	Increased peripheral circulation	Administer medication as prescribed
		Follow procedure to ensure safe administration of intravenous medication
		Monitor vital signs according to protocol
Reduced mobility	Supports are in place to facilitate day-to-day activities provision of appropriate mobility and	Refer patient to physiotherapist and occupational therapist for assessment and home aids
	Patient able to maximize mobility safely	Ensure all aids are accessible
		Assess for home care support for day-to-day activities
		Arrange supports as necessary
Patient at risk of developing pressure sores	Tissues remain free from pressure sores	Complete a standardized pressure risk assessment
		Provide appropriate pressure relief equipment to meet individual needs
		Avoid shearing, tearing and friction forces
		Ensure the patient's position is frequently and safely changed
		Protect dry and cracked skin using a non-allergenic emollient
		Encourage mobility and a nutritious diet
Loss of sleep	The patient is well rested	Relieve pain and reduce anxiety. Ensure the environment is conducive to the patient's needs
Anxiety	Reduced anxiety	Assess need for counselling and refer as appropriate
	Supports in place	Allow patient time to express his/her concerns Listen to patient sympathetically in a relaxed environment
		Provide as much information as possible to enable patient to make informed choices
		Allow patients to be as active in the management of their care as they feel able
		Provide relatives with the support and information they need to help the patient

Angioplasty is often performed on the same occasion as an arteriogram, which indicates the position and length of the stenosis. Its success is dependent on:

- the ability of the catheter to pass through the stenosis
- the length and position of the stenosis
- the ability of the balloon to stretch the lumen of the vessel and crack the atheromatous plaque
- adequate remodelling of the lumen
- the compliance of the patient in following a healthy lifestyle.

In the 1980s, laser-assisted angioplasty was introduced to recanalize peripheral arterial vessels. The idea behind this was to allow the laser beam to burn into the atheromatous occlusion. Although this method has met with a mixed response, nurses need to be aware that it is an option (Ford 1990).

Complications following angioplasty

Possible complications are as follows:

- thrombosis
- embolus
- haematoma formation and haemorrhage
- rupture of the vessel wall
- allergic reaction to the radiographic medium or anaphylactic shock induced by the radiographic medium
- arrhythmias
- cerebrovascular accident
- dislodgement of calcified plaques, which become lodged more distally and result in further distal occlusion
- false aneurysm due to perforation of the vessel wall (this is rare).

Nursing management

Before the angioplasty

- It is important to ensure that the patient is fully informed of the situation. He or she will need to understand why the procedure is being undertaken and what the potential outcomes are. Explaining that resting on the bed after the procedure will reduce the risk of haemorrhage from the puncture site will aid compliance.

- The radiologist will require information about the patient. It is necessary, therefore, to ensure that all documentation, including informed consent for procedure, medication chart and information regarding any known allergies, goes to the radiography department with the patient.

- Recording the patient's blood pressure, pulse, respiration and temperature prior to the procedure will provide sound baseline observations that will serve as a reference for post-angioplasty monitoring.

- Starving the patient for 6 hours prior to the procedure will allow an emergency embolectomy to be carried out if necessary.

- In some centres, removal of hair from the procedure site may be requested. An antiseptic solution will be applied by the radiologist prior to insertion of the cannula.

After the angioplasty

- Nursing care and monitoring will follow the same routine as for patients undergoing angiogram (see Ch. 5).

- Health promotional advice needs to be reinforced before the patient's discharge; if necessary, this can be followed up by agencies in the primary care sector. For example, the patient may benefit from the support of smoking cessation groups. The promotion of exercise will encourage the development of a collateral circulation to enhance tissue perfusion.

- Aspirin may be prescribed as antiplatelet therapy where there is no known adverse reaction.

- Owing to the usual process of wound healing, as described in Chapter 2, a smooth intimal lining is promoted. The stenosis may reform as a result of intimal hyperplasia.

CONCLUSION

In the longer term, if it is not possible to control the symptoms of vasospastic and small vessel disease, patients may require amputation in order to enjoy a better quality of life.

For patients with chronic major vessel disease, exacerbated by an acute episode, bypass reconstructive surgery is beneficial in 70% of cases. It is therefore often worth attempting, in spite of the risks, since it holds out the hope of a better quality of life for these patients.

REFERENCES

Ernst E 1991 Peripheral vascular disease, benefits of exercise. Sports Medicine 12(3): 149–151

Ernst E, Matrai A 1987 Intermittent claudication, exercise and blood rheology. Circulation 76(5): 1110–1114

Ford K A 1990 Laser-assisted angioplasty in the patient with peripheral arterial disease. Journal of Vascular Nursing 8(3): 6–8

Forrest A P M, Carter D C, Macleod I B 1985 Principles and practice of surgery. Churchill Livingstone, Edinburgh

Fowkes F G R, Housley E, Riemersma R A et al 1992 Smoking, lipids, glucose intolerance and blood pressure as risk factors for peripheral atherosclerosis compared with ischaemic heart disease in the Edinburgh Artery Study. American Journal of Epidemiology 135: 331–340

Green C 1993 Anti-streptokinase titres after topical streptokinase. Lancet 341: 1602–1603

Green M A, Shearman C P 1994 Reperfusion injury in peripheral vascular disease. Vascular Medicine Review 5: 97–106

Hallett J W Jr, Brewster D C, Clement Darling R Jr 1995 Handbook of patient care in vascular surgery, 3rd edn. Little, Brown, Boston

Kannel W B, Shurtleff D 1973 The Framingham study: Cigarettes and the development of intermittent claudication. Geriatrics 28: 61–68

Larsen A O, Lassen N A 1966 Effect of daily muscular exercise in patients with intermittent claudication. Lancet 2: 1093

Leng G C, Fowkes F G R 1993 The epidemiology of peripheral arterial disease. Vascular Medicine Review 4: 5–18

LeMaitre G, Finnegan J 1980 The patient in surgery: a guide for nurses. Saunders, Philadephia

Vowden K R, Vowden P 1996 Peripheral arterial disease. Journal of Wound Care 5(1): 23–26

Jamieson E, McCall J M, Blythe R 1992 Guidelines for clinical nursing practices related to a nursing model, 2nd edn. Churchill Livingstone, Edinburgh

Palatini P 1988 Blood pressure behaviour during physical activity. Sports Medicine 5: 353–374

Paul M C, Halfman-Franey M 1990 Laser angioplasty in peripheral vascular disease. Critical Care Nurse 10(5): 65–78

Caring for the patient with critical ischaemia, undergoing reconstructive bypass surgery

In 1981, it was determined by a working group at the Vascular Symposium held in London that it is necessary to have a clearly defined definition of *critical ischaemia*, in order to reconcile the differences of opinion on the efficacy of the wide range of surgical interventions and therapies available for treatment. If clinical trials of therapy are to be considered reliable, patients need to be clearly categorized. No definition can encompass every patient group that presents with critical ischaemia. Therefore patients presenting with diabetic disease should not be included, as any coexisting neuropathy and the high risk of infection can skew ischaemic signs and symptoms. Only those falling into the clearly defined categories discussed below should be considered as presenting with *critical ischaemia*:

1. Acute ischaemia.
2. Chronic ischaemia with an acute episode.

Critical ischaemia is defined as 'A limb suffering from acute, or acute progression superimposed imposed upon chronic ischaemia, which requires urgent surgical intervention to improve its circulation' (Jamieson et al 1982).

> **Appearance of the ischaemic limb**
>
> • cyanosis
> • mottling
> • pallor
> • dependent rubor
> • pallor on elevation
> • shiny, hairless skin.

ACUTE ISCHAEMIA

This was defined by the International Symposium of Vascular Surgeons in 1981: 'A limb which suffers acute arrest of its circulation, which had previously been normal, may be defined as suffering from critical ischaemia when there is persistent objective evidence of motor or sensory loss'. An objective measure may be considered to be an ankle pressure of less than 40 mmHg, or less than 60 mmHg with superficial tissue necrosis of the foot or digital gangrene to the level of the base of the toe (Jamieson et al 1982) (Fig. 9.1). The latter part of this definition was subsequently changed by the Modified International Symposium Working Party to read simply: 'tissue necrosis or digital gangrene irrespective of the ankle pressure'.

However, a European working group definition includes severe rest pain for at least 2 weeks *or* ulceration or gangrene *and* ankle artery pressure of less than 50 mmHg (Tyrrell & Wolfe 1993).

Today fewer patients present with acute ischaemia because of the decrease in the incidence of rheumatic heart disease; this used to be complicated by atrial fibrillation, which is a potent source of arterial emboli.

> Critical ischaemia is a state in which a limb is at risk of being lost. This may result from:
>
> • an acute episode
> • an acute on chronic episode
>
> Objective indications are:
>
> ABPI < 40 mmHg or < 60 mmHg with tissue necrosis.

ACUTE ON CHRONIC ISCHAEMIA

In the presence of long-term occlusion of that which is less than critical, a further relatively small acute insult may arise and provoke critical ischaemia as described above.

Those patients with arterial ulcers, gangrene or rest pain alone do not fall into the 'acute on chronic ischaemia' group but into the group with chronic ischaemia, as discussed in Chapter 8.

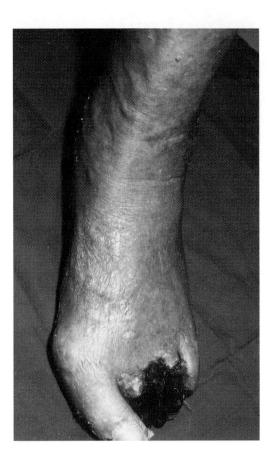

Fig. 9.1 Digital gangrene.

With increasing intensity of ischaemic symptoms in the lower limbs, associated with atherosclerotic arterial occlusive disease, peripheral aneurysm, thrombosis and arterial thromboembolism, patients' quality of life will deteriorate. Thirty years ago patients may well have faced primary amputation to alleviate their discomfort, but, with advances in technology and surgical techniques, today's critically ischaemic patient has the opportunity to avoid this. However, if there is evidence of irreversible ischaemia, as indicated by fixed skin mottling or induration and necrosis of muscle, the prognosis may be too poor for urgent revascularization to be considered, and it may not be possible to save the limb.

With the critically ischaemic patient, for whom a conservative management programme, angioplasty or fibrinolysis have failed to improve perfusion, embolectomy or reconstructive surgery—depending on the cause of occlusion—may well be indicated. However, consideration will need to be given to the general medical and cardiopulmonary status of the patient, given the risk of anaesthesia and surgery. The status of proximal inflow vessels and distal run-off vessels is also significant if reconstructive surgery is to be considered; if these are grossly diseased, a bypass will be of questionable benefit.

Nursing this patient group is challenging, as many present with a complex of coexisting vascular and associated problems. Coronary or carotid disease, hypertension and cerebrovascular disease, renal occlusive disease and diabetes are not uncommon. Some may present with vasculitis or haemolytic disorders, and many will have endured claudication for many years and experienced high levels of pain and fear. Some may still be the breadwinners of the family or have dependents to care for. Aspects of lifestyle may well have contributed to their lower limb ischaemia, and old habits die hard.

Pre-admission health promotion and support will greatly improve the outcome of bypass reconstructive surgery by reducing the risk of chest infections related to smoking, and of infection associated with obesity and a poorly controlled diet. Promotion of exercise within the limits of the individual's capacity will enhance recovery. All these issues will need addressing if one is to reduce the risk of postoperative complications.

ASSESSMENT

A careful *history* will be required. This will document any episodes or previous signs and symptoms of peripheral vascular disease, including carotid arterial disease and cardiopulmonary disease. The familial incidence of these and any known disease such as diabetes should be noted, as should risk factors such as poor nutrition, obesity, high stress levels, smoking and high alcohol intake.

A history of fractures, bone deformities and disease such as arthritic disease may interfere with postoperative mobility, and an awareness of these disorders is helpful. Consideration needs to be given to the condition of the skin, especially where patients will be lying on a theatre table for around 4 hours, as pressure risk scores may be high in the ischaemic patient. Skin which has become thin and has the appearance of tissue paper may not respond well to adhesive dressings applied at the end of surgery. Any history of allergies should be brought to the attention of everyone involved with the patient.

Presentations in arterial occlusive disease

Arterial occlusions are most commonly found at the bifurcation of vessels where blood flow is most turbulent, or along the lumen of the superficial femoral and distal vessels; carries the *threat of limb loss*.

Tissues may display *discoloration* such as cyanosis, mottling, extreme pallor, or dependent rubor which changes to pallor on elevation. The skin may appear shiny and hairless and toenails may be thickened and ribbed owing to the poor perfusion of nutrients.

> • Minor loss: resting ankle pressure < 60 mmHg with monophasic Doppler reading. Clinically non-healing ulcer and/or focal gangrene.
> • Major loss of tissues: flat Doppler wave form.

In the presence of microembolic occlusion, painful *patchy cyanotic areas* may present, particularly in the plantar regions of the feet and on the toes—these could be mistaken for bruising. Cardiac disease, aneurysms or distal thrombus are common sources of microemboli.

Ulceration, commonly found on the foot, is a classical sign of arterial insufficiency. Where the patient presents with critical ischaemia, these ulcers will normally fail to heal unless perfusion can be restored.

There may be areas of *necrosis and gangrene*, particularly on the tips of the toes. Infection is evident if the gangrene is wet with blisters and blebs of pus. The presence of *Clostridium welchii* will cause gas gangrene.

> Differential diagnosis from ischaemic pain
>
> • osteoarthritis
> • diabetic neuropathy
> • neurogenic pain
> • Sudeck's atrophy
> • venous claudication.

Pain

Critically ischaemic pain needs to be differentiated from pain caused by osteoarthritis, diabetic neuropathy, neurogenic claudication caused by spinal stenosis, Sudeck's atrophy and chronic venous insufficiency.

> Levels of pain
>
> • intermittent claudication
> • rest pain
> • rest pain and tissue loss.

The position of pain, its duration and association with other symptoms will be an indicator as to the cause. A classical symptom is the need to hang the foot/leg out of the bed at night to relieve the pain.

However, the cascade of pain (see Ch. 8) is an indication of the degree of occlusion. In critical ischaemia one would expect that the patient had reached *category 3: tissue loss in the presence of severe rest pain and nocturnal pain.*

> Use of the cascade concept of degree of pain will help to define degree of occlusion.

MANAGEMENT OF THE PATIENT WITH ACUTE THROMBOEMBOLIC CRITICAL ISCHAEMIA

It is difficult to distinguish immediately between a thrombotic and an embolic episode. In the absence of previous peripheral vascular disease, an incident is more likely to be associated with an embolus than with a thrombus.

An embolus may occlude any of the major arteries, and signs will be those associated with any sudden ischaemia to the vital organs affected:

- cerebral and vertebral arteries: CVA
- superior mesenteric artery: ischaemia of the small intestine
- renal artery: acute ischaemia of the kidney
- femoropopliteal artery: ischaemia of the lower limbs
- axillobrachial artery: acute ischaemia of the arms, hand or digits.

Investigations

A full past medical history and assessment of the presenting symptoms will suggest the possible diagnosis of arterial embolus.

Depending on the site involved, investigations may include:

- chest X-ray
- electrocardiogram
- abdominal ultrasound
- arteriography
- computed tomography
- urinalysis
- Allen's test
- blood screening
- Doppler ankle brachial pressure index and assessment of pedal pulses.

Treatment

This should be implemented at the earliest possible time to reduce the risk of long-term hypoxic damage to tissues. Once the diagnosis has been made, an initial infusion of heparin should be administered, as this will reduce the risk of distal and proximal thrombosis.

Conservative management

Fibrinolysis

Fibrinolysis is the process by which fibrin in thrombus is broken down by fibrinolytic (thrombolytic) agents, without recourse to surgery.

There are three agents in common use. *Streptokinase* is produced from beta-haemolytic streptococcus group B; *urokinase* is derived from renal tissue cultures; and *alteplase (rt-PA: tissue type plasminogen activator)* occurs naturally as a secretion of vascular intimal cells. They all act to convert plasminogen to plasmin, a proteolytic enzyme, which breaks down fibrin.

> Fibrinolysis: the process by which thrombus is broken down using fibrinolytic agents such as:
>
> - alteplase (rt-PA)
> - streptokinase
> - urokinase.

Streptokinase is relatively cheap, but has the disadvantage of provoking severe allergic reactions, even anaphylaxis, especially on repeated use, as antibodies are formed. Therapy must, therefore, not be repeated within 6 months. Concern has been raised in relation to the topical use of streptokinase, which is found in enzymatic products for débriding wounds. Although no connection between the use of topical streptokinase in wound management and anaphylaxis has been made, titres of anti-streptokinase antibodies were found to be raised in all of five patients in a small study by Green (1993). The recommendation is, therefore, that topical streptokinase should only be used in patients with a low risk of myocardial infarction who are unlikely to require systemic streptokinase.

Urokinase is more expensive but less likely to cause allergy. rt-PA is nonallergenic, being a natural substance, but is the most expensive agent.

Applications

Most commonly, these agents are used in the early treatment of coronary thrombosis in acute myocardial infarction, or in severe pulmonary embolism. Urokinase tends to be used for ophthalmic embolic disease. As far as the vascular patient is concerned, use is indicated for acute arterial graft occlusion, blockage of central venous pressure lines, or acute arterial thrombosis. Some clinicians extend their use to the treatment of recent, extensive DVT, other arterial occlusions—especially if surgery is contraindicated or if a thrombus is inaccessible—or even acute stroke. Fibrinolytic agents may be used with caution in combination with heparin and/or aspirin.

Fibrinolysis carries less risk for patients than do anaesthesia or surgery, particularly given the chance of postoperative myocardial infarction. Also, it will not damage the underlying normal vessel structure, such as the valves in veins. Sometimes fibrinolysis and angioplasty are combined, as the agents, particularly rt-PA, may effectively shorten the thrombus beforehand.

The half-lives of the agents are short, particularly that of rt-PA (5–8 min), so continuous infusion over several hours is often necessary.

In the vascular patient lesions less than 7 days old tend to respond better to thrombolysis than longer-lasting lesions. Administration may be i.v. via volumetric pump, or intra-arterially via angiogram catheter. The catheter may be passed through the thrombus and slowly the thrombolytic agent is infused.

Alternatively, *pulse spray fibrinolysis* has recently been developed. In this procedure, which is carried out in the radiology department, a catheter with several eyelets along its length is introduced into the thrombus, and the fibrinolytic agent is infused by pressure pulses.

Contraindications to treatment are situations where bleeding might occur, namely pregnancy, menorrhagia, surgery within the last 10 days, a history of peptic ulcer or oesophageal varices, cerebrovascular bleed or diabetic retinopathy. However, these contraindications are all relative, as the treatment may be life (or limb) saving. A balance has to be drawn. Liver disease and a known allergy to the agents being used may also contraindicate therapy.

Streptokinase is antagonized by tranexamic acid should bleeding occur. However, *rt-PA has no antidote*.

Nursing management

• One should ensure that a complete drug history is taken, especially for antiplatelet drugs or anticoagulants. Enquiring about recent streptococcal infections is recommended before using streptokinase, as these may reduce its efficacy.

- The patient should have had a full clotting screen and blood count, and have had blood cross-matched.
- Tranexamic acid and steroids (for anaphylaxis) should be at hand.
- The patient should be monitored closely for haemorrhage from the puncture site and from that of any recent surgery, especially if this procedure is undertaken to relieve thrombus formation in a recently implanted graft. Vital haemodynamic signs should be continuously monitored.
- Haemoglobin and fibrinogen levels should be monitored to pick up occult bleeding from overtreatment.
- The limb should be observed at frequent intervals for colour, temperature and the presence of a pulse on Doppler ultrasound examination. Reperfusion will be demonstrated by improved Doppler signals and resting ankle brachial pressure index.
- Bed rest during the procedure will help to prevent haemorrhage being induced at the puncture site through movement. A downward tilt on the foot of the bed will aid peripheral vascular perfusion.
- The administration of analgesic medication as prescribed will help to reduce discomfort from pain.
- Relief of pressure from any ischaemic limb, whether caused by the weight of the limb against a surface, by shearing or by friction, will help to prevent pressure-sore development and enhance patient comfort.
- Bed cradles may be supportive in relieving the weight of bed linen, but care needs to be taken to ensure that ischaemic limbs are not knocked against the frame.
- If there is surface bleeding, direct pressure needs to be applied. Likewise, the application of pressure on removal of the infusion catheter will reduce the risk of haemorrhage.
- Protocols for the administration of intravenous infusions should be implemented in order to reduce the risk of microorganisms entering the circulation.
- Having time to listen and respond to patients' anxieties will help to reassure them, especially where this improves their understanding of their situation. It is important to maintain the balance between support and hope, on the one hand, and the risk that fibrinolysis may be unsuccessful and result in the need for surgery on the other.
- The patient can expect an angiogram at the end of treatment, and this procedure should be explained. The results should be given to the patient by a member of the medical or radiological team, and nurses have an important role to play in improving patients' understanding.
- The patient may be allowed to eat and drink following the insertion of the catheter for fibrinolysis, but it is wise to check first with the medical team.

Anticoagulation

Anticoagulants are given either intravenously or orally. The intravenous anticoagulant of choice is usually *heparin*. Indications for the use of heparin are similar to those for the fibrinolytic agents, but in situations that are less acute or life-threatening. Standard heparin is used as an i.v. treatment for abnormal clotting, as it has a strongly negative charge and high affinity for antithrombin III. It is also given to flush intravenous lines during an operation where temporary anticoagulation is required, and in situations where oral anticoagulant has not yet reached a stable level. It is the anticoagulant of choice in pregnancy, as the oral drugs may produce deformities in the fetus, and standard heparin's large molecular size prevents it from crossing the placental barrier.

A low-molecular-weight version of the drug has been developed, and this can be given subcutaneously twice a day, as it has a longer half-life. It acts differently from standard heparin, as it inhibits clotting factor X, making it useful for the prevention of DVT (see Ch. 6). The antidote to all heparin is i.v. protamine sulphate, 1–1.5 mg/100 units heparin.

Contraindications and side-effects are mostly related to the risk of bleeding, as for fibrinolytics. Hypersensitivity to heparin can occur, and caution should be observed in hepatic and renal disease. Heparin can cause thrombocytopaenia.

Oral anticoagulants include coumarins such as warfarin and phenindione. Warfarin is by far the most common drug of choice.

Warfarin is convenient and has a fair margin of safety for use at home. However, it takes 3–5 days to achieve adequate anticoagulation because the clotting factors it affects have longish half-lives. Heparin is given concurrently if the need for anti-coagulation is urgent. Similarly, clotting tests remain abnormal for up to 5 days after the drug has been stopped. Activity is measured by use of the INR (see Ch. 5).

Side-effects again revolve around bleeding problems. In addition, warfarin may cause skin necrosis, patches of dark-looking degenerating skin that can appear in any site—often the breasts, buttocks and arms. This slowly resolves when the drug is stopped.

Warfarin interacts with a large number of drugs which serve to enhance its effect by displacing it from its binding protein and thereby increasing the proportion of free warfarin in the circulation. (Codeine does not do this, and therefore is the only safe analgesic for patients on warfarin, unless the level of analgesia is constant, allowing the maintenance of a constant INR at the new dose.) Stopping or starting such drugs can seriously increase the risk of bleeding. They include aspirin, non-steroidal analgesics, dextropropoxyphene (as in co-proxamol) and even long-term high-dose paracetamol. Other drugs which enhance the effect of warfarin are tetracyclines, carbamazepine, dipyridamole, oestrogens, cimetidine and, importantly, alcohol. Drugs which reduce the effect of warfarin are some antibiotics, including erythromycin, co-trimoxazole, ciprofloxacin and metronidazole.

This list of less commonly used drugs is not exhaustive, so if in doubt always check with the *British National Formulary*.

Phenindione can be used as an alternative, for patients who are hypersensitive to warfarin.

The antidote to warfarin is *fresh frozen plasma* for a rapid effect, or *vitamin K*, which is active within 6–12 hours. It may take up to 2 weeks before heparin is effective again after the administration of vitamin K, whereas it is immediately active again following the use of fresh frozen plasma.

Surgical Management

Embolectomy

Preparation

• The patient is prepared for theatre in the normal way.
• Blood will be cross-matched and saved.
• The infusion of heparin should be discontinued 6 hours prior to surgery to reduce the risk of haemorrhage; it can be reversed if necessary.

Intra-operatively

• A cut-down procedure is performed to allow the insertion of a Fogarty embolectomy catheter, with which the embolus is removed.

- An on-table angiogram will show whether the occlusive matter has been completely cleared.
- The vessel is then closed.

Post-procedure
- The patient will be observed for haemorrhage and changes in haemodynamic status.
- The colour, warmth and the presence of Doppler ultrasound arterial signals will be monitored.
- Echocardiography will establish whether there is any remaining debris in the right atrium.
- The patient may be discharged with antiplatelet or anticoagulation medication such as aspirin or warfarin.

Bypass surgery

Bypass surgery can greatly enhance the quality of life and prevent the loss of a limb for patients presenting with critical ischaemia or severe claudication.

Investigations

Patients may undergo some of the necessary investigations as outpatients, or they may be admitted to hospital for a few days.

A resting ankle brachial pressure index of less than 0.8 denotes ischaemia. However, where the ABPI is less than 0.5, the disease is significant enough to warrant consideration of surgical intervention. The recording of segmental pressures is useful in determining the level of occlusion.

Useful investigations are as follows:

- Angiography is the most definitive investigation that can be performed to establish the position and extent of the blockage in the blood vessels (Fig. 9.2).

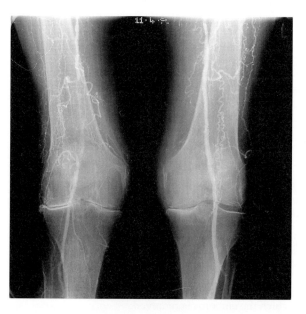

Fig. 9.2 Angiogram.

- *Digital subtraction angiography* will produce conclusive information regarding the best site for proximal inflow and distal outflow. One needs to establish that there is sufficient inflow and distal runoff to support a graft before deciding that reconstruction is a feasible option. The measurement of flow is more important than angiography results in predicting whether surgery will have a successful outcome (Stirnemann et al 1994).

- A *duplex scan* may be required to assess the calibre of the saphenous or brachial veins and to determine the feasibility of autologous reconstruction surgery. A duplex scan may also be performed just prior to surgery to map the position of the veins.

- *Blood tests* will include a full blood count, creatinine, urea and electrolytes, lipid levels, group and cross-matching (usually for at least 4–6 units of blood), and coagulation tests (including screening for antithrombin III, as a deficiency of the latter may lead to postoperative arterial thrombus formation).

- An *electrocardiogram (ECG)* will identify previous myocardial infarction or cardiac arrhythmias, which could put the patient at risk of cardiac dysfunction or embolus generation.

- A *chest X-ray* will routinely be requested to assess the patient's suitability for anaesthesia, and may detect the presence of thoracic aneurysms.

- *Respiratory function tests* may be called for if the patient presents with coexisting pulmonary disease.

- *Baseline recordings* of blood pressure in both arms, the quality, rhythm and rate of the radial pulse, temperature, rate of respiration and status of pedal pulses, including ABPI, will all be beneficial in assessing the postoperative stability of the patient's condition. The condition, temperature and colour of the skin should be observed.

- *Ward urinalysis* should be mandatory to eliminate the presence of glucose, ketones, protein, infection or specific gravity levels outside the normal range.

- *Blood glucose tests* should be performed at ward level if the patient is known to be diabetic. Ward blood sugar tests will be recorded to meet the individual management needs of each patient.

- *Cognition* needs to be evaluated in order to ensure that there is informed consent and to enable staff to give patients information that will allow them to contribute positively to their own recovery. It is important that patients understand the risk factors involved in surgery, and that this has been communicated to their family and to significant others without increasing anxiety. The positive outcomes of surgery need to be emphasized. The long-term patency rates (3 years and over) vary from 80% for a vein graft to a proximal artery to 55% for an expanded polytetrafluoroethylene (ePTFE) graft to a distal vessel. With ongoing graft surveillance and early intervention the life of a graft can be extended.

Revascularization will unfortunately not be successful for some patients, who will then require amputation. The immediate success or otherwise of bypass surgery is generally recognized within the first 5 postoperative days.

A *full nursing assessment*, including day-to-day activities, psychosocial aspects, ethnic and spiritual issues and the need for social services to provide home support, will be made on admission. The individual needs of the patient must be determined and communicated to members of the multidisciplinary team.

Nutritional and hydration status needs to be evaluated pre-operatively. The patient may well have had a restricted diet owing to high levels of pain that have led to poor mobility, loss of appetite and anxiety. Any special diets, such as high protein, diabetic and ethnic, will need to be highlighted. Diabetic patients need a sliding scale insulin regime.

Pressure relief assessment, which will allow the provision of equipment and appropriate nursing intervention to ensure that pressure is sufficiently relieved, has to be a high priority. In distal disease of the limbs, patients will be particularly prone to pressure sores on their heels, and an ongoing assessment needs to be made to enable measures to be taken to avoid this. The use of bed cradles will alleviate pressure on ischaemic limbs.

Pain should be assessed and managed according to individual needs. Tilting the foot of the bed down may aid perfusion and reduce pain. Analgesic medication needs to be monitored for its effectiveness and titrated accordingly. If constipation is a side-effect of the analgesia, a laxative may be required.

Anxiety level assessment will help to ensure that patients are at ease in their new environment and that they feel able to discuss any anxieties with carers. Patients may need to be given additional information about postoperative management and appropriate lifestyle.

Preparation for theatre

Local protocols regarding the preparation of patients for theatre will be followed. A pre-operative shave may be required 24 hours before surgery. Recording height, weight and nil by mouth for a 6-hour period prior to surgery is normally mandatory.

> It is important to consider the pros and cons of obtaining consent for amputation at the same time as consent for bypass.

Alderson et al (1994) underline the important role nurses have in helping the patient to understand what doctors are saying about the proposed surgery prior to signing a consent form. Nurses are responsible for safeguarding the interests of individual patients in accordance with the UKCC guidelines (UKCC 1989) and they need to ensure that the patient has a clear understanding of exactly what surgery is to be undertaken. Unfortunately, it can happen during bypass reconstruction surgery that the procedure for which consent was given is not feasible and that amputation is inevitable. If this has been taken into account beforehand, and the patient has consented to bypass reconstruction surgery or amputation if necessary, the latter procedure is then permissible under the one anaesthetic. However, not all patients are able psychologically to make this decision for fear that they will lose a limb which may otherwise have been revascularized. To do the surgery in two operations has the disadvantage that two anaesthetics are needed and that the patient faces disappointment for a second time as he or she watches the bypass surgery fail. Nurses can lend support to patients in making important decisions about consent.

> The nurse has an important role in helping patients to understand what is said about their need for surgery, prior to giving consent.

It is not uncommon for patients undergoing reconstruction surgery to be catheterized in the anaesthetic room, as this will avoid discomfort in the early postoperative phase.

Conventional reconstructive surgery

The technique of inserting a graft proximal to an occlusion and securing it distally allows tissues to be revascularized. The collateral systems carry blood to the tissues in between the proximal and distal ends of the bypass graft (Fig. 9.3).

> It is necessary to rely on collaterals to carry blood to tissues that are in between the proximal and distal ends of a graft.

Revascularization may be performed using an in situ autologous vein graft stripped of its valves and harvested from the leg, arm or umbilicus. If this is not possible a synthetic graft made from expanded polytetrafluoroethylene (ePTFE) or dacron may be used, as illustrated in Figure 9.4.

If revascularization is to be performed using an autologous vein, this will be harvested first through intermediate incisions along the length of the leg. Great care is needed in order not to damage the epithelium of the vessel, and poor surgical technique during this part of the procedure may result in skin flap necrosis.

Having established pre-operatively the position of the occlusion and which vessels are most suitable for reconstruction bypass surgery, the surgical team makes

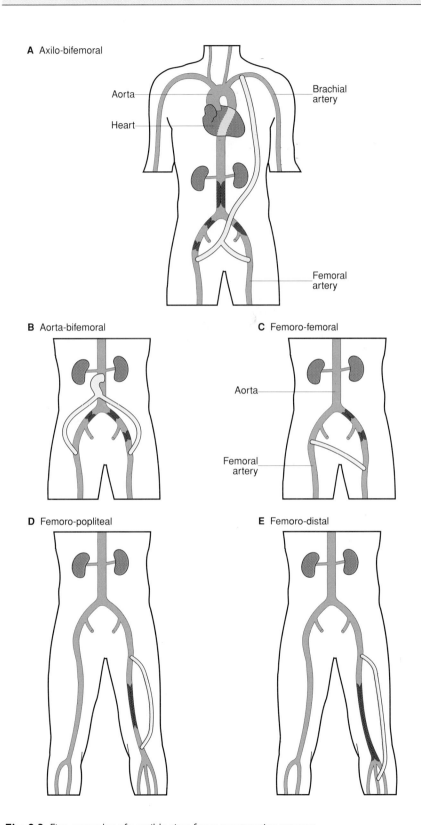

A Axilo-bifemoral

Aorta

Heart

Brachial artery

Femoral artery

B Aorta-bifemoral

C Femoro-femoral

Aorta

Femoral artery

D Femoro-popliteal

E Femoro-distal

Fig. 9.3 Five examples of possible sites for reconstruction surgery.

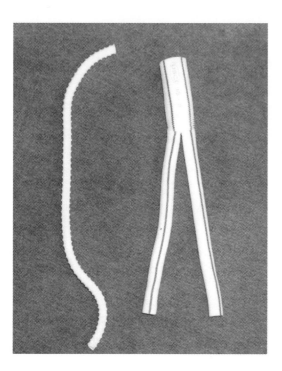

Fig. 9.4 Samples of synthetic graft—ePTFE and dacron.

an incision proximal to the occlusion and attaches the graft to the vessel. The graft is then tunnelled under the skin to a point distal to the occlusion, and anastomosed to the vessel there. Discrepancies between the decreasing size of the lumen of distal vessels and the diameter of ePTFE grafts, or between the lumen of an autologous vein and that of the femoral artery, may be accommodated by specialized surgical techniques such as the use of a Miller cuff. On-table angiography and a Doppler perfusion assessment will be performed prior to skin closure to check for technical errors (Fig. 9.5)

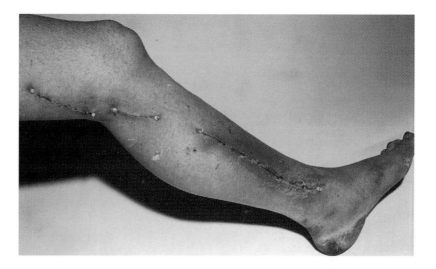

Fig. 9.5 The wound in a patient who has undergone a femoral distal bypass.

Postoperative management

To permit continual monitoring it is usual after the operation for patients to go to a high-dependency unit or to intensive care until they have stabilized.

Patients who presented with severe disease at the popliteal trifurcation and distal vessels carry a higher risk of postoperative myocardial infarction or cerebrovascular accident than those with superficial femoral artery disease (Quinones-Balrich & Caswell 1991). Close monitoring is required for the first 48 hours and oxygen as prescribed should be administered. This has the double function of helping to reduce the incidence of myocardial infarction and helping the patient to recover from the anaesthetic gases.

Continual routine haemodynamic monitoring will be required in the early postoperative period until the patient has stabilized. Specific attention will be given to monitoring colour, the skin temperature of the foot, and the presence of pedal arterial pulses (by the use of Doppler ultrasound). The Doppler signal may be graft-dependent and therefore only found in the reconstructed vessel if the remaining distal vessels are diseased. Hourly Doppler assessment will alert staff early to the possibility that the graft is failing and may facilitate effective early intervention in the form of embolectomy or reconstruction of the graft.

> Postoperative graft surveillance by means of hand-held Doppler ultrasound will allow intervention at the earliest possible time should the graft show signs of failing.

As the patient becomes stabilized the frequency of observations can be reduced.

An intravenous infusion will remain in place until the patient is eating and drinking and as long as intravenous antibiotics are required. Prophylactic antibiotics will help to reduce the risk of infection.

In the early postoperative weeks, the reconstruction vessels will not have a blood supply from the vasa vasorum. Should they become infected, antibiotic therapy is unlikely to be effective. Synthetic grafts carry a higher incidence of failure resulting from infection than do autologous grafts.

The groin is a common site for infection, especially in obese patients whose skin folds rub and become moist from perspiration. Attention to hygiene, especially in the skin folds of the groin, will help reduce this risk. Talcum powder should be avoided. It is important to place urinary catheter tubing away from the surgical incisions. Haematoma formation can be a source of infection, and therefore may necessitate evacuation. The use of a drain for the first 24–48 hours will help to eliminate the risk of haematoma formation. Strict aseptic technique has to be maintained during the management of dressings and care needs to be taken to avoid irritation of the incisional lines.

> The groin is a common site for infection, and one should therefore:
> - promote diligent skin hygiene between skin folds in the groin
> - avoid talc
> - site urinary catheter tubing away from the area
> - identify and evacuate haematomas
> - use an aseptic technique when managing wounds.

Observation for haemorrhage and haematoma formation is important. It should not be allowed to go unnoticed simply because it is obscured by the bed linen, as there may be considerable loss of blood in a very short period of time. The loss may go unrecognized by the patient who remains sedated from the anaesthetic; and, because blood is at the same temperature as the body, bleeding may not always be felt immediately. In such cases, collapse may be the first indication that haemorrhage is occurring.

In the event of haemorrhage, pressure should be applied above the site of anastomosis rather than directly onto it, since this will protect the graft. Medical help should be summoned immediately and plasma expanders infused as prescribed until a blood transfusion can be administered.

Causes of graft failure

Causes of graft failure and thrombus formation can be identified as technical and non-technical (Table 9.1).

Postoperative lower limb oedema

Reperfusion oedema The sudden increase in hydrostatic pressure alters the balance against the osmotic pressure, resulting in an increase in extracellular fluid. It

Table 9.1 Causes of graft failure

Technical	Non-technical
Poor construction of the anastomosis	Inadequate inflow/outflow
	Friability of distal vessels
Vein graft too small	to which the graft has been anastomosed
Compression from extrinsic muscle or tendon	Hypercoagulation
Kinking of the graft	Overzealous activity in the first postoperative days
Intimal flap elevation	Haemorrhage due to breakdown in the anastomosis
Clamp injury	
Poor technique when harvesting the vein graft	Formation of haematoma
	Introduction of infection
	Rejection of synthetic graft

- Post-surgical inflammation is a common feature following reconstructive surgery; in moderation this is acceptable
- Compartmental syndrome = extreme inflammatory oedema → muscles in fascia unable to expand → ischaemia due to high pressure → nerve entrapment → trauma → fasciotomy.

takes from 6 weeks to several months for the body to adjust to reperfusion, and oedema may remain for this period of time. Oedema can be reduced by leg elevation, gentle exercise and compression hosiery once the wound has healed, providing the postoperative ankle brachial pressure index has improved.

Surgical inflammatory oedema Postoperatively, the inflammatory response to surgery may result in oedema, particularly in the popliteal space and calf. Should mobilization occur too soon, pressure from this will be placed upon the wounds and may compromise healing or dislodge the skin closures. Bed rest for 3–5 days may be required. Avoiding knee flexion will help to prevent inflammatory oedema from compromising the wound. Elevating the foot of the bed slightly may also help to reduce the swelling.

Compartmental syndrome

Acute ischaemia produces inflammatory oedema, which may be extreme. The muscle groups of the calf are encased in tight fascia which cannot expand; therefore, if ischaemia is allowed to continue for more than 8 hours, the pressure within the muscle compartments can cause irreversible tissue damage. Damage to nerves that pass through the compartments may also arise. Fasciotomy is sometimes required, and some surgeons may do this prophylactically if complete occlusion occurred more than 6 hours before surgery.

Careful monitoring of calf measurements, sensation and pedal pressures may help to alert the surgeon to the need for medical intervention to prevent permanent tissue damage.

Reperfusion injury

When an acute occlusion in a limb is suddenly relieved, further damage can occur. There are a number of reasons for this. Oxygen forms radicals which can destroy cell membranes, resulting in the release of the metabolites of anaerobic respiration. Myoglobin, a substance found in muscle that is responsible for intramuscular aerobic respiration, is also released. In addition, capillaries can become blocked on reperfusion, in accordance with Coleridge's 'white cell trapping theory' (Thomas et al 1988, Coleridge-Smith et al 1988). This is described as the 'no reflow' phenomenon, which stops fresh blood reaching the tissues. According to Burnard's theory, fibrin is laid down along the capillaries, so occluding the vessel pores and preventing diffusion (Burnard et al 1982). The systemic effects can be severe. The breakdown of muscular cell membranes produces hyperkalaemia and myoglobinaemia, with the products of anaerobic respiration predisposing the patient to acidosis.

Local symptoms of reperfusion injury include pain from oedematous swelling, which may lead to compartmental syndrome as described above. Muscle weakness and difficulty in moving the limb may be experienced.

The technique of gradual reperfusion at a slow rate is also beneficial peri-operatively after release of the obstruction to avoid the above.

It is possible to measure compartment pressure on the ward by the insertion of a needle attached to a transducer. The normal pressure should be nil; but if the pressure has risen to the level of the patient's diastolic pressure, ischaemia occurs.

Treatment considered may include reducing the extent of reperfusion injury by perfusing blood which is low in white cells, or by administering fibrinolytic agents. However, bleeding is a complication of the latter procedure, particularly as this is taking place as a postoperative procedure. Fasciotomy may be undertaken to relieve the above.

Treating possible systemic effects urgently is essential as myoglobin precipitates in the kidneys and may cause renal failure. Monitoring the colour of the urine for the presence of the characteristic brownish hue and for high specific gravity should be undertaken at frequent intervals. Hourly fluid balance should be maintained.

Regular blood samples are required for analysis of myoglobin levels, urea and electrolytes, and creatinine.

Systemic treatment requires the maintenance of sufficient blood volume and pressure, particularly to the kidneys. Dobutamine to maintain blood pressure can be used effectively. Diuretics are also used to increase urine output.

Hyperkalaemia is managed using insulin and glucose, and acidosis by using a carefully monitored infusion of sodium bicarbonate. Finally, pain relief is usually required.

Despite these measures, the mortality rate from reperfusion injury varies from 15% to 40% and that of subsequent amputation is 20% (Quinones-Balrich & Caswell 1991).

Reperfusion injury
Sudden reperfusion results in occlusion:
• oxygen forms free radicals
• to destruction of cell membranes and metabolites of anaerobic respiration are released
• plus release of myoglobins
• to microcirculatory congestion
• to 'no reflow' phenomenon
Therefore:
• breakdown of muscle cells
• hyperkalaemia
• myoglobulinaemia
• acidosis
Results in:
pain, swelling, muscle weakness.

Anxiety

It is not uncommon for patients who have had a bypass to feel a high degree of anxiety in the early postoperative days as they will be concerned to know that the graft has taken and that they are not going to require amputation. A positive response and attitude to stress can enhance hormonal balance and immune response, which are compromised by negative responses (Simonton 1978). Patients need time to ask questions and should be given open and honest replies. It may take several days before it is known how well the graft has taken. Diversional therapy such as listening to music or watching television, and pursuing passive hobbies, such as embroidery, painting, word puzzles, reading and conversation with others in the ward can all help to pass the time.

Pain

This needs to be managed to meet the individual's needs (See Ch. 4).

Pressure sores

Care of pressure areas must be ongoing for all ischaemic patients. Pressure points will be under considerable strain during the peri-operative period and in the first postoperative days whilst bed rest is enforced. Oedema may further reduce the perfusion of oxygen to tissues. The behaviour of patients who are tense or fearful of moving will put them at greater risk of pressure sore formation. All these issues need to be addressed to ensure continuing prevention of pressure sores. The use of a monkey pole over the bed may help the patient to move without causing friction or shearing of tissues.

Ongoing nursing management

Clothing It may be more comfortable for male patients to wear shorts postoperatively, as this will reduce discomfort along incisional lines and enable close observation of the wound site, whilst retaining the patient's dignity.

A *nutritious* diet should be encouraged as soon as the patient feels able to eat and drink, to promote wound healing.

In order to *reduce the risk of trauma in the first postoperative day,* bed rest is normal. Passive leg exercises need to be encouraged and, unless contraindicated, patients will be anticoagulated to reduce the risk of DVT. As the oedema reduces in the foot/ankle, on the second or third postoperative day, the patient may sit in a chair with the leg elevated.

Patients need to be given the opportunity to *discuss their anxieties* about the success of the surgery and may need much reassurance until they are secure that adequate reperfusion has been achieved, eliminating the need for amputation.

By the third day, the *intravenous infusion, urinary catheter and wound drain should all have been removed,* allowing the patient more ambulatory freedom. Whilst encouraging mobility, it must be balanced with adequate rest to allow healing and reduce the risk of oedema increasing. *Elevation of legs* should be maintained whilst the patient is resting. *Standing should be avoided.*

The *wound* will need to be *carefully monitored* for blistering, haematoma formation or bleeding. The use of tape on the skin is to be discouraged as this may traumatize fragile tissues. It is essential that infection is not allowed to enter the wound and healing is promoted without the wound becoming sloughy or necrotic.

Where the wound has become sloughy or necrotic and lies over a synthetic graft, the application of topical wound care products to remove slough will need to be done with caution. The graft may lie just below the slough and the use of desloughing agents containing propylene glycol may have adverse effects on the impermeability of the synthetic material, should they come into contact, resulting in leakage from the graft.

Skin closures are normally removed around the 17th postoperative day, depending on wound healing.

It is essential for patients to pay attention to personal hygiene. In the first postoperative days they may need assistance with this, as washing, etc. has to be carried out from the bedside. Provided the wound is dry and healing well, showering or bathing is acceptable by the fifth postoperative day and will help to reduce the risk of infection by the removal of debris in which microbes thrive. However, it is not advisable for patients to soak for too long, as this may soften tissues and make them susceptible to infiltration of pathogens. (See Sample Clinical Guidelines, p 180–182.)

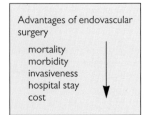

Advantages of endovascular surgery

mortality
morbidity
invasiveness
hospital stay
cost

Endovascular reconstructive surgery

This form of surgery is still in its infancy, but the use of stents, inserted under radiological control, is less invasive than conventional methods. At present its use is confined to patients with more minor symptoms and shorter stenoses. Such operations have a lower mortality and morbidity, require a shorter stay in hospital and cost less than conventional surgery (Becquemin et al 1995).

Discharge from hospital

Patients may well be discharged from hospital on low-dose aspirin to reduce the risk of platelet aggregation and thrombus formation. They should be made aware of the importance of lifestyle, as this is essential to preserving the patency of the graft and maintaining adequate perfusion. Arterial disease is never confined to one segment of the body, and realizing the implications of an unhealthy lifestyle may convince patients of the need to be careful.

On discharge patients must be advised to contact the hospital or their general practitioner *immediately* if they experience any unusual symptoms in the limb, such as excessive coldness or a difference in temperature from the contralateral limb, numbness, cramp, excessive pins and needles, discoloration or pain. Teaching the patient or his family how to palpate pedal pulses will give them a better idea of when they should seek urgent medical help.

It is not uncommon for those who have undergone popliteal distal reconstruction surgery to feel a tightness in the popliteal space, or for those who have had any form of reconstruction surgery to feel the graft below the skin. Patients need to know that this is normal. Advice regarding the signs of wound infection, general malaise and pyrexia should also be given to patients.

Matters such as driving, exercise, work, sexual activity and relaxation should all be discussed with the patient prior to discharge. Patients' information leaflets are useful for reinforcing the information given on discharge, since there is much that patients have to take on board as they leave the security of the ward environment; having an information leaflet to refer back to, and a contact number to call, will help to build confidence.

The community nurse may be requested to oversee wound healing and remove skin closures. She or he will provide ongoing professional supervision and the support required to meet patients' ongoing needs.

CONCLUSION

With advances in vascular laboratory facilities across the country, graft surveillance programmes are reducing the incidence of amputation. Establishing protocols for the early detection of graft failure and the need for intervention has been found to be more cost-effective for this patient group than resorting to primary amputation (Cheshire & Wolfe 1993). By keeping them under surveillance and offering further surgical intervention, should it be required and technically possible, one can offer such patients a more active quality of life.

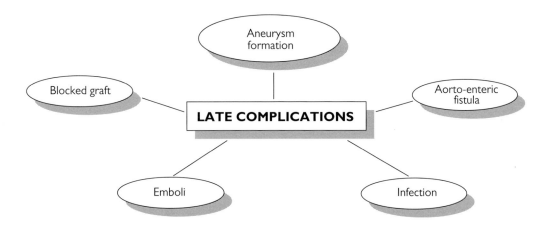

Fig. 9.6 Late-onset complications of reconstruction surgery.

The ethics of selecting patients for bypass surgery depending on their ability to adopt a healthier lifestyle and stop smoking needs consideration. The NHS is working with limited resources and there are many patients who require reconstruction surgery. Should the medical profession be selecting patients on the basis of lifestyle, family dependants and age? Is it valid to consider that poor compliance will inevitably lead to future degenerative arterial disease and possible graft failure?

SAMPLE CLINICAL GUIDELINES FOR THE CARE OF PATIENTS UNDERGOING BYPASS RECONSTRUCTIVE SURGERY

Bypass check list

Action	Date	Signature
Pre-operative care		
Patient admitted to the ward either as a planned admission or via the emergency department. Criteria—ABPI < 0.5, intolerable pain, gangrene, or extensive tissue loss.		
(If planned admission, the patient is advised to bring in a pair of short pyjamas or night shirt as this will enable easier management post-operatively.)		
Angiogram should demonstrate adequate inflow and runoff vessels.		
Vital signs are recorded as baseline observations, ensuring the blood pressure is recorded in both arms to avoid missing any alteration due to calcification or stenosis of the brachial arteries.		
ABPI should be recorded in all distal vessels to establish baseline observations.		
Nursing assessment of activities of daily living are recorded.		
Any allergies or special needs are noted.		
Height and weight are recorded in the nursing documentation.		
Pressure sore risk is assessed and appropriate provision of resource to prevent pressure sore should be established.		
A pain monitor is implemented and analgesia titrated to provide comfort.		
Tip down the foot of the bed to assist arterial perfusion to distal vessels.		
Repeat angiography should be undertaken if not already performed.		
Blood screening—FBC, U&Es, ESR, coagulation screen cross-match 6 units.		
Chest X-ray, ECG, and echogram if required.		
The multidisciplinary team members are alerted to the patient's admission.		
Discharge planning is commenced.		
Informed consent to anaesthesia and surgery is made.		
Patient is prepared for theatre.		
Twenty-four hours pre-operatively, the groin and leg are shaved if requested by the surgical team. This may be performed by either the patient or carer.		
The patient must be nil by mouth for 6 hours pre-operative.		
Angiograms, notes and prescription chart must go to theatre with the patient.		

Cont'd

Bypass check list (cont'd)

Action	Date	Signature

Postoperative care

Continually monitor vital signs in a high dependency area for 24 hours.

Observe the limb for ischaemia, by monitoring colour, temperature and the presence of Doppler ultrasound signal when checking distal pulses. (NB: the limb may be graft dependent and therefore a signal may be present in only one distal vessel. It is important to establish the details of surgery performed when evaluating the patient's progress postoperatively.)

Use oxygen as prescribed and regular oxygen saturation assessment.

Observe for postoperative haemorrhage or haematoma.

Maximize patient comfort by ensuring adequate pain control is maintained through the administration of prescribed drugs. In the presence of patient controlled analgesia, ensure the patient fully understands how to manage their pain control. Follow local guidelines for the care of a patient with a PCA or epidural.

Measure and record redivac drainage every 24 hours.

When drainage has subsided, the redivac should be removed as soon as possible at the surgeon's request to avoid infiltration of infection.

All wound drainage tubing should be kept away from urinary catheter drainage tubing.

Observe fluid balance.

Ongoing care of the patient with a urinary catheter introduced to avoid creating any discomfort to the patient by necessitating them to use urinals/bedpans or commodes in the first 2 postoperative days.

Care of the patient with a cannula and intravenous infusion.

Free fluids and diet as tolerated once fully conscious.

Ongoing management after the first 24 hours

Ongoing monitoring for haemorrhage at the wound site (should haemorrhage arise, manual pressure should be applied to the limb, above the level of the graft insertion).

Ongoing monitoring for graft occlusion leading to ischaemia using Doppler ultrasound, observation of skin colour or temperature. Inform medical staff of any critical incident.

Ongoing monitoring for graft infection.

Administer prescribed drugs, including antibiotics.

Ongoing pain assessment and titration of analgesics as prescribed to maximize patient comfort.

Monitoring and recording of vital signs reduced over the forthcoming days to 4 hourly, tds, bd then daily if within normal limits.

Providing access is not required for intravenous antibiotics, the patient is accepting fluids and diet to maintain hydration and nutrition, the intravenous infusion will be discontinued.

The urinary catheter is removed after 48 hours providing the patient is able to pass urine without discomfort.

Ongoing care to prevent pressure sores.

Ongoing care of the patient to prevent deep vein thrombosis. (Anti-embolic stockings should only be applied on direction of the surgeon and should not be applied where the ABPI is less than 0.7.)

Cont'd

Bypass check list (contd)

Action	Date	Signature
To prevent reperfusion oedema, legs should be elevated and level with the hips whenever the patient is sitting down. Passive leg exercises should be encouraged.		

Mobility — 1st postoperative day — up for bed making only
— 2nd postoperative day — may sit in a chair with legs elevated
— 3rd postoperative day — short walk only to the toilet
— 4th postoperative day and onwards — gently increase mobility.

Hygiene—Patients should be given assistance as required, with special attention to ensuring the groin remains clean, dry and free from particulates (including talcum powder).

Providing the incision line has fused together, a shower or bath may be considered after the 3rd day.

Skin closures are removed around the 14th–17th day at the discretion of the surgeon.

Arrangements for this will need to be made within the primary nursing team if the patient is to be discharged before this time.

Discharge

Low-dose long-term aspirin may be prescribed along with any other medication to take home.

The patient will need to be aware of the arrangements for ongoing wound management and removal of skin closures.

Advice should be given regarding elevation of legs when sitting to reduce reperfusion oedema.

Ongoing health promotion advice should be given with a view to reducing the risk of further arterial disease.

The patient should be encouraged to take a daily walk as far as possible, within their individual capability.

An outpatient follow-up appointment date should be given to the patient.

The patient should be advised that at this time they may have a duplex scan in order to survey the graft patency and this may be routinely repeated if they are included in a graft surveillance programme.

The patient should be advised to seek medical help immediately should they experience any signs of ischaemia in either leg, breakdown of the incision line, infection or excessive pain, or if they feel unwell in any way. It is important that they do not wait until the follow-up appointment should they experience any of the above.

Driving should not be recommended until they are able to perform an emergency stop and therefore it is better to wait for at least 4 weeks post operation.

Sexual activity may be recommenced after 2–3 weeks providing the patient feels happy about doing so.

Any individual patient needs and resourcing which require input from social services and other members of the multidisciplinary team, should be in place on discharge.

REFERENCES

Alderson P et al 1994 Women's view of breast cancer treatment and research. Social Science Research Unit, London

Becquemin J et al 1995 Conventional versus endovascular surgical procedures; a no choice option. European Journal of Vascular and Endovascular Surgery 10(1): 1–3

Burnard K et al 1982 Pericapillary fibrin in the ulcer-bearing skin of the leg; the cause of lipodermatosclerosis and venous ulceration. British Medical Journal 285: 1071–1072

Cheshire N J W, Wolfe J H N 1993 Critical limb ischaemia: amputation or reconstruction. In: Wolfe J (ed) ABC of vascular diseases. BMJ Publications, London

Coleridge-Smith P D et al 1988 Causes of venous ulceration; a new theory. British Medical Journal 296: 1726–1727

Green C 1993 Antistreptokinase titres after topical streptokinase. Lancet 341: 1602–1603

Jamieson C W et al 1982 The definition of critical ischaemia of a limb. British Journal of Surgery 69(Suppl): S2

Quinones-Balrich W J, Caswell D 1991 Reperfusion injury. Critical Care Nursing Clinics of North America 3(3): 525–534

Simonton C, Simonton S 1978 Getting well again. Tarcher, New York

Stirnemann P et al 1994 Intraoperative flow measurement of distal run off; a valid predictor of outcome of infrainguinal bypass surgery. European Journal of Surgery 160(8): 431–436

Thomas P R S et al 1988 White cell accumulation in dependent legs of patients with venous hypertension; a possible mechanism for topical changes in the skin. British Medical Journal 296: 1693–1695

UKCC 1989 Exercising accountability: a framework to assist nurses, midwives and health visitors. UKCC, London

FURTHER READING

Keller I, Bzdek V 1986 Effects of therapeutic touch on tension headache pain. Nursing Research 35(2): 101–105

Krieger D 1972 The response of in-vivo human haemoglobin to an active healing therapy by direct laying on of hands. Human Dimension 1: 12–15

Krieger D et al 1979 Therapeutic touch; how to use your hands to help or heal. Prentice-Hall, Englewood Cliffs, NJ

Pasquinelli G et al 1990 Healing of prosthetic grafts. Scanning Microscopy 4(2): 351–362

Rutherford R B et al 1986 Suggested standards for report dealing with lower extremity ischaemia. Journal of Vascular Surgery 4(80): 1986

Taylor R S et al 1992 Improved technique for polytetrafluoroethylene bypass grafting: long term results using anastomotic vein patches. British Journal of Surgery 79: 348–354

Tyrrell M R, Wolfe J 1993 Critical leg ischaemia; an appraisal of clinical definitions. British Journal of Surgery 80: 177–180

Caring for the patient undergoing amputation

Amputation of a limb should be considered as a positive way of ensuring that a greater quality of life can be enjoyed than that with which patients have been coping to date. Most have been suffering high levels of pain and immobility. The decision to amputate will only be taken when there are no other options left open.

The prevalence of amputation is 1.3 per 1000. 75–80% of amputees are over the age of 60, and the incidence is greater in men than in women, with a ratio of 3:1. This is steadily levelling out to a ratio of 3:2.

Epidemiological studies demonstrate that the number of lower limb amputees referred to limb-fitting centres each year is between 500 and 1000 per million population. The amputee population in England is around 52 000 lower limb and 11 000 upper limb amputees—a total of 63 000. The prognosis following amputation for ischaemic disorders is poor: nearly a third of unilateral leg amputees lose the other limb within 3 years and half of them will die within 5 years.

Peripheral vascular disease accounts for 63% of amputees. Ischaemia results from occlusion caused by atherosclerotic disease, calcification of vessels and thromboembolus, Buerger's disease, inflammation of vessels and vasospastic disorders. Ischaemia leads to a lack of diffusion of nutrients and oxygen from the peripheral circulation to the tissues, resulting in cell death. Extreme pain is experienced and, if left untreated, the ischaemia will result in gangrene and possible systemic illness (septicaemia), which may even lead to death.

Other causes of amputation are diabetic disease (22%), trauma (6%), malignancy (3%), infection (2%) and deformity (1%) (McColl 1986) (Fig. 10.1).

The patient may already be in hospital, and so be familiar with carers and the ward routine, since amputation is sometimes needed following orthopaedic surgery, or bypass surgery where the patient has rejected a graft. In these cases patients will already be known to the professionals caring for them, and some of the pre-operative investigations and interventions may not be required.

Alternatively, where the patient was clearly unsuitable for reconstruction surgery, a conservative management programme may have been implemented in order to maximize the period of time before amputation became essential.

However, some patients are not known to nursing and medical professionals until the situation is too late for conservative surgery, and therefore they present as emergencies requiring immediate amputation.

> The majority of lower limb amputees are:
> - male
> - over 60
> - patients with peripheral vascular disease.

> Over 20% of amputations are for diabetic disease.

INFORMED CHOICE

Taking the decision to agree to amputation will be made easier for patients if they have an understanding of what to expect after the operation—physically, emotionally and psychologically. Informing them of the services and supports which will be brought in to assist them in maximizing their mobility and independence will help to relieve anxiety. Consenting to the operation and anaesthetic often takes a lot of courage, and helping the patient to make an informed choice is critical in aiding his or her acceptance of the need for surgery.

Owing to the confusion and general malaise resulting from the heavy analgesia

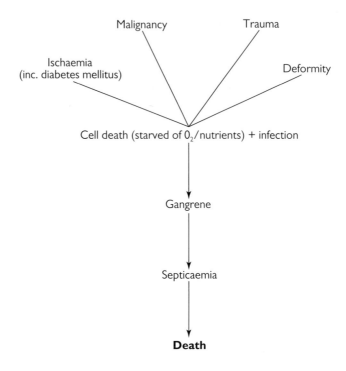

Fig. 10.1 Causes of amputation.

needed to keep them comfortable, and the toxins associated with a gangrenous limb, patients may not always be in a position to make a rational decision for themselves regarding the need for surgery. The final decision will then be the surgeon's responsibility. This decision is normally made after discussion with the family.

PROFESSIONALS INVOLVED

Multidisciplinary involvement with the amputee:

- nurse
- doctor
- physiotherapist
- occupational therapist
- social services
- prosthetist
- counsellor
- disablement resettlement officer
- dietician

In order to give patients as much independence as possible, many professional people will be involved in their care, offering support and advice and helping them to come to independent decisions. It will help patients if they know who is to be involved in supporting them in their treatment and on the road to recovery and independence. If it is possible, meeting members of the multidisciplinary care team before the operation will enhance patients' sense of security and trust and give them an opportunity to ask questions. A multidisciplinary approach will enable patients to make informed choices and take control of their own future, at a level on which they and their relatives feel able to manage.

The nurse

The nurse has an important role to play in ensuring that the patient's situation is communicated to other members of the multidisciplinary team, which may include clinicians, physiotherapists, occupational therapists, prosthetists, counsellors, dieticians, social workers and disablement resettlement officers. Members of the multidisciplinary teams work closely together, offering clinical care and psycho/social support. Nursing intervention should be aimed at promoting the recovery of the patient and sound wound healing.

The occupational therapist

The overall aim of the occupational therapist is to help the patient, as an individual, to maintain a satisfactory quality of life. The therapist will carry out a home assessment, so ensuring that the environment into which the patient is to be discharged is safe, and that he or she can safely attend to personal hygiene needs, has appropriate toileting facilities, and can get to the toilet and move from one area of the house to another safely. These factors are important in maintaining self-esteem. Alterations to doorways and steps and the installation of stair lifts may be necessary, and the occupational therapist will assess the individual's needs in these areas and liaise with social services for the provision of facilities.

In many centres it is the responsibility of the occupational therapist to order wheelchairs. Early acquisition of a wheelchair does help to encourage independent mobility and gives the patient the opportunity to learn the skills of manoeuvring in a supported environment.

A *pre-operative wheelchair assessment* will ensure that the correct width of wheelchair is ordered. Bilateral amputees require set back wheels and support to cope with the altered centre of balance that follows the loss of both limbs. Measuring the patient's height and weight will guarantee that the wheelchair is the correct size. Wheelchairs are made in different shapes and sizes, but generally a chair which has large front castors and set back wheels is less likely to tip backwards. It is designed so that the back tilts slightly backwards to accommodate the new centre of gravity and helps to prevent the patient from feeling as though they are falling forwards. The foot steps need to be adjusted to enable the patient to rest his foot/feet comfortably on it without overbending his knees. The arms of the chair should be at a comfortable height, and it is essential to check that the brakes are in full working order. Trays can be fitted to the front of the chair to help patients carry items. Training patients to manoeuvre wheelchairs will be the responsibility of all professionals caring for them, but in the main it will fall to the occupational therapist to see that they can move safely over different surfaces. Where a lot of time will be spent in a wheelchair, it is important to ensure that a pressure relief cushion is also ordered. Transporting a wheelchair may cause a problem if carers do not have a car that will accommodate one; they may therefore need to make arrangements to acquire a suitable vehicle.

Stump boards for below-knee amputees will need to be added to the wheelchair to support the limb in an extended position in order to reduce the risk of flexion contractures.

Slide boards, used to enable transfer from one seat to another, and monkey poles can all be ordered pre-operatively. The early assessment of needs will enable one to acquire the necessary resources in good time and reduce the risk of delays on discharge. If equipment is in place, rehabilitation can be started without delay, allowing patients' self-esteem to be built up before frustration and demoralization set in.

The physiotherapist

Physiotherapists help the patient achieve mobility. Getting to know the physiotherapist before the operation will enable the patient to be positively aware of ways in which physiotherapy can help towards his or her recovery.

Pulmonary function assessment and postanaesthesia deep breathing and expectoration techniques will help to reduce the risk of postoperative chest infections.

Being introduced to active exercises designed to strengthen the limbs and reduce the risk of postoperative deep vein thrombosis will help patients understand what the physiotherapist requires of them postoperatively in both the acute and rehabilitative phase of their recovery.

The dietician

The dietician may be asked to give patients advice. Wound healing will be dependent on a well balanced diet. Where patients present with special dietary needs related to individual tastes, cultural expectations or medical requirements, dietetic involvement is warranted. Patients may present as malnourished. High levels of pain may lead to them becoming anorexic or unable to purchase the items needed to maintain a well balanced diet. A diet rich in protein, iron, calories and vitamins A, C and D is essential for recovery.

The energy expenditure of a normal-limbed person walking on the level at 70–75 m/min has been calculated as 59 cals/min/kg. So it follows that an 80-kg man walking at this speed for half an hour would use up just over 140 000 cal or 140 kcal.

The use of a prosthetic limb will increase calorific demand, and therefore the appetite must be stimulated and calorific intake raised to meet this increased demand, as shown in Table 10.1.

Social services

Social services may also be brought in if patients require alterations to the home in order to accommodate their changed mobility status. The provision of additional support at home, in the form of home care, emergency call lines or meals on wheels, will need to be assessed pre-operatively so that services can be implemented at the earliest possible time and delays avoided on discharge.

Amputees who are still working will benefit from a referral to the *disablement resettlement officer*, who will be able to give advice regarding new skill training schemes and assist in finding a new job, should this be necessary.

The support of a *trained counsellor* may help patients to come to terms with amputation. This need may not be recognized by patients while they are in the protected environment of the ward, but a contact for counselling support can prove invaluable in meeting the emotional needs of a patient after discharge. The contact should be aware of patients' fears and frustrations. Coming to terms with an amputation may take a patient through all the stages of bereavement. For those who are breadwinners or carers within a family there are added concerns regarding their responsibilities; making the necessary adjustments to accommodate the need for support is not always easy, and may lead to feelings of guilt, failure or frustration.

REFERRAL FOR PROSTHETIC LIMBS

To suggest that a limb can be fitted is not always realistic, and may build false hopes. Therefore one needs to make a careful holistic assessment of general health,

---

Disability benefits

Under 65:
• care allowance
• mobility allowance

65 and over:
• attendance allowance.

Table 10.1 The percentage increase in daily calorific intake needed for different levels of amputation

Level of amputation	% calorie increase
Single below-knee	10–40
Double below-knee	40 +
Single above-knee	60–65
Double above-knee	65 +
One above and one below knee	200: 3 times normal calorific expenditure
Wheelchair	9

mobility and mental status before deciding to refer for a prosthesis. For many people, a prosthetic limb can prove to be more of a hindrance than a help. For example, a female has to remove the limb every time she needs to use the toilet. Where patients have coexisting disease such as severe arthritis, poor mobility or congestive cardiac failure, limb fitting is not always the answer: it is sometimes kinder to help patients come to terms with the possibility of being independently mobile from a wheelchair (Fig. 10.2). However, if it is possible to make a referral for a prosthetic limb, the prosthetist who has technical expertise, will ensure that the prosthesis is matched to the needs of the individual.

Patients may also derive benefit from *gait assessment*. Referrals can be made to gait laboratories where data can be collected using video footage and lightweight instruments that can be incorporated into footwear insoles (goniometers). These devices are placed over the joints and connected to a small unit worn on a waist belt which transmits information to a computer data bank. The information collected is used to determine the forces and pressures exerted on the lower limbs during walking. This measurement of joint and muscle function can be used to aid and monitor further treatment in order to ensure that patients are not putting abnormal pressures on joints and thus causing damage to healthy tissues in the long term. Correct gait and stance can enhance self-esteem and make the prosthesis less conspicuous. Incorrect gait may lead to abnormal pressures on other areas of the body, resulting in muscle strain and bone deformities. Table 10.2 highlights some gait deviations.

Patients presenting with any of the signs given in the table should be referred immediately to the prosthetist for prosthetic adjustment and to the physiotherapist and gait technician for assessment and support. Skin on the stump, the ischial tuberosity and the remaining leg and foot should be checked for cracks, pressure sores or signs of rubbing. It is worth enquiring whether the patient has changed the height of shoe heels, as this will upset the correct balance. Patients need to be

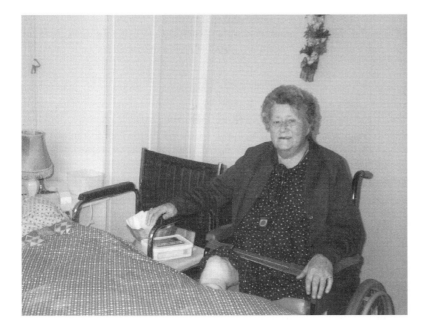

Fig. 10.2 A bilateral amputee successfully managing at home.

Table 10.2 Gait deviations

Gait deviation	Presentation
Abducted gait	Prosthesis appears to give discomfort in the groin Contracted abductors Feeling of insecurity, therefore walks with a wider base Prosthesis appears too short
Lateral trunk bending	Short stump and/or weak abductors Lack of support to femur from lateral socket wall Prosthesis appears too long Inability to hip hitch
Circumduction	Uneven step length Habit
Vaulting	Inability to extend hip over prosthesis during the stance phase as a result of hip flexion contracture or weak extensors
Uneven timing	Reluctance to bear weight on prosthesis owing to discomfort or insecurity Prosthesis too long
Uneven arm swing	Uneven step length combined with a very short stance phase on prosthesis Pain on ischial seating Fear and insecurity Weak hip extensors Poor balance Lack of balance Lack of confidence Habit

reassured and praised, without being patronized, for their attempts to become mobile. This will build their confidence and keep up their spirits.

The gait and clinical measurements team will include a *bioengineer, a consultant in rehabilitation medicine, a prosthetist, an orthotist and a physiotherapist.*

PAIN

Pain by itself can be extremely debilitating, resulting in lack of sleep, tension, exhaustion and emotional distress. The aim is to keep patients free from pain at all times and reduce the incidence of postoperative phantom pain or sensation.

Phantom pain/limb sensation

The cause of phantom pain and sensation still baffles scientists, but it is recognized that there is an association between physical and psychological factors. Astill (1993) suggests that 'The physical theories are associated with the physical organs or part of the body, for example, the nerve supply and nerve endings'. This is because the brain retains a map of the body as it was. The ends of nerves which used to run from the amputated area need time to settle down and adjust to the body's new map. Sometimes this fails to happen, and the patient experiences intractable pain, even when attempts are made to divide the nerves higher up. Nerves attempt to regenerate from their cut ends and when they have no limb to travel down they can form into nodules called neuromas. Unfortunately, removing a neuroma only allows a new one to form.

The psychological theories suggested by Astill (1993) are that 'An individual's basic personality, thoughts and emotional responses are connected to the presentation of phantom phenomena'. Sociocultural influences will also have a bearing on the degree of phantom sensation experienced.

Management of phantom sensation and pain will need to address these issues effectively. All adult patients who have undergone amputation will imagine that they can still feel a part of the body which has been removed or feel discomfort in this region. The degree to which they experience these sensations will depend on the individual and on the *level of pain control before the operation*. Children experience less phantom sensation.

Sensations may be associated with movement that reflects movement in other parts of the body. For example, the phantom may appear to stretch as the patient yawns. Itching, temperature changes, pressure and touch may all be sensed. Phantoms may be willed or be a spontaneous sensation of movement. They can remain very vivid for 2 to 3 years after surgery and then become less real—shorter and less intense—as time goes by, though in some cases they can last for life.

Phantom pain needs to be distinguished from stump pain and other less common causes of pain such as osteomyelitis, ischaemia and bony spurs, as any of these can be experienced. Phantom pain in the early postoperative phase is often described as knife-like or lancing. In the ensuing years this changes to become a sensation of burning, squeezing, cramping, crushing, aching, stabbing or a distorted sense of the position of the phantom limb. Twitching of the muscle in the stump may accompany phantom pain. Though phantom pain will diminish over a period of several years, weather changes, stress and tension, autonomic actions such as elimination, yawning and stretching may all aggravate fluctuations in the pain (Sedgwick 1993).

Patients should be made aware that phantom pain and sensation are a normal postoperative feature so that they are able to accept and come to terms with them in a realistic way.

Placing furniture on the side of the patient which is not to be amputated will help to ensure that he or she learns to lead with the remaining leg, so reducing the risk of a distressing outcome. The patient should be advised not to lead with the stump and not step back on a phantom limb if he or she is using crutches or a frame and is not wearing a prosthesis.

Controlling pain

Pain is a subjective experience and is individual to each person. To state that it is inevitable in this patient group can only serve to reduce the quality of care received by patients. It is not supportive to minimize the effect pain may be having on patients by being too dismissive in attempting to help them psychologically to come to terms with the need for amputation. One school of thought advocates keeping pain control to a minimum, because masking pain will delay the patient's acceptance of surgery. The other school of thought believes that pain control must be maximized and every effort made to ensure comfort and a reduced risk of postoperative phantom pain and sensation.

Adequate pain control pre-operatively will help to reduce phantom pain. It is important to ensure that the patient knows that he or she should inform the staff if pain control is inadequate.

Ongoing review and titration of analgesia, as prescribed, needs constant attention. Pain may be assessed using a standardized form.

Drugs may be given orally or by injection, at regular intervals. Delayed-release morphine sulphate tablets, twice daily, are often the analgesic of choice. This can be titrated with morphine solution 2-hourly or as prescribed for breakthrough pain. Alternatively, patient-controlled analgesia (PCA) or continuous lumbar infusion may be used; this ensures that there is continuous pain relief, so reducing the risk of postoperative phantom pain/sensation. With PCA it is usual to give oxygen via a mask or nasal specs to complement the drugs in the infusion. Amitriptyline has also proved effective when used in conjunction with morphine and can reduce the sensation of postoperative phantom pain. Carbamazepine may be prescribed to reduce the frequency of these nerve impulses.

Alternative therapies for pain control may be considered. Gentle massage and tapping of the stump may help the brain to adjust to the new situation and reduce phantom sensation. Where nurses or patients have specialized knowledge of aromatherapy and are qualified to practise this, massage with appropriate aromatic oils may prove helpful. The soothing effect of reflexology or acupuncture, administered by a qualified person, also has its place.

Physiotherapists may suggest the use of a TENS (transcutaneous electrical nerve stimulation) machine, which is a small, battery-operated device that can be worn unobtrusively by the patient and has small pads attached to the skin. It is thought that the electrical stimulation promotes the release of endorphins, which relieve the pain, and also stimulates nerve fibres, which compete with the pain impulses, thereby tending to block them. This is explained in the discussion on the Gate theory in Chapter 4. They may also provide intermittent pulse spray therapy (mega pulse) to aid pain control.

It is helpful to tilt the foot of the bed down to aid the arterial perfusion of blood and oxygen to the lower limbs. A bed cradle, which keeps the weight of the bedclothes off the ischaemic limbs, will also help to relieve pain.

Patients may not be able to deal, psychologically, with the urgent need for surgery, but, given adequate counselling and knowledge of what is happening physiologically, they can be supported in coming to terms with the inevitability of amputation at the earliest possible time. Ethically one must ask which is the kindest way forward for the individual patient.

HEALTH PROMOTION

As stated in Chapter 3, it is important that the patient should be as fit as possible prior to surgery.

PRE-OPERATIVE INVESTIGATIONS

If the patient has already had failed bypass or orthopaedic surgery, much of the pre-operative picture will already be in place. However, should he or she present as an emergency, a chest X-ray and ECG will be performed. Blood will be screened for urea and electrolytes, a full blood count, group and save.

Recording the patient's weight and height before the operation will help the occupational therapist obtain the correct wheelchair in good time.

Pre-operative monitoring of haemodynamic status, respiratory status and core temperature will provide a baseline measurement against which to assess the stability of the patient in the postoperative period.

Suitability for anaesthesia will be assessed by the anaesthetist. Where there are cardiopulmonary problems, amputation under a spinal block may be considered the safest option.

Where diabetes is a known factor, blood sugars need to be recorded regularly in the ward, and urine should be tested for glucose and ketones. The latter, if present, could be indicative of a metabolic ketoacidosis, especially where the patient has become anorexic owing to systemic toxicity, anxiety and pain.

Sliding scale insulin may be required pre-operatively if the patient has become toxic. This may be continued during and after surgery until the condition has stabilized and a normal diet is being tolerated.

If the patient has been anticoagulated, the warfarin will need to be discontinued prior to surgery and a continuous infusion of unfractionated heparin commenced.

Consideration will need to be given as to both the most appropriate level of amputation and discharge needs. This decision should be made at a case conference of members of the multidisciplinary team. Any muscle weakness, arthritis or cardiopulmonary difficulties are noted and communicated to members of the team. The peripheral vascular status of the other limb and any coexisting disorders, for example malignancy, should also be taken into consideration.

If a prosthesis is used the myocardial oxygen demand will increase by 60%, and adequate pulmonary function therefore will need to be demonstrated. Assessment with a peak flow meter will help to ascertain the functional level.

The provision of a monkey pole over the bed will help to relieve pressure on the sacrum, if correct usage is demonstrated. It will also help with toileting while patients are bed-bound. After the operation, because of the change in the centre of gravity, simple movements such as sitting up and turning over become more difficult. Patients should aim to become familiar with the monkey pole pre-operatively, so that by the time of the operation its use will have become habitual.

Pre-operative use of passive leg exercises reduces the risk of thrombosis in the good leg, and deep breathing will help to reduce the risk of chest infection after surgery. Pre-operative practice will automatically enhance postoperative activity. In the first few days emotional distress and the weakness resulting from surgery may reduce the patient's concentration in cooperating with the new therapies being promoted.

If pain is reasonably well controlled pre-operatively, other exercises to strengthen limbs and muscles not previously used in mobilization and balance can be practised. For example, active exercises to strengthen the arms with blocks on which to press up, lifting the buttocks off the bed, pushing the back of the knee into the bed, and lying supine will all help to strengthen limbs postoperatively and reduce the risk of flexion contractures. Patients should be advised not to hold the stump in flexion. Maintaining good posture, holding in the buttocks, standing tall and keeping the stump vertical when standing will all promote successful postoperative rehabilitation. Patients with below-knee amputations should be made aware that holding the stump in flexion at the knee may result in contractures that will make it difficult to fit a prosthesis.

A standardized tool should be used to assess pressure sore risk, and the appropriate equipment for pressure relief should be obtained in order to forestall pressure sore development. This is a high-risk patient group, as the vascular disease will already be contributing to poor tissue oxygen perfusion, and nutrition and mobility may be low owing to high levels of pain.

If patients are unable to elevate themselves off their sacrum, nursing intervention at frequent intervals to alleviate pressure is essential, even if a pressure relief mattress is being used.

Early referral to a social worker for the assessment of needs and implementation of supports—for example, meals on wheels, home care and alterations to the patient's accommodation—will help to speed up the patient's discharge. The social worker will also be able to give advice regarding financial benefits such as:

- attendance allowance or disability allowance for patients under the age of 65.
- a mobility allowance and the acquisition of disability car stickers to facilitate parking.

Driving may not always be feasible postoperatively, but it is something which needs to be discussed in order to help patients maximize their independence. Cars can be adapted to enable amputees to continue driving; the addresses of useful contacts who can give further information about this can be found in Appendix 1 at the end of this book.

If appropriate, early referral to a rehabilitation centre will alert specialists in this field to a patient's need for postoperative assessment and possible support. Early referral will hopefully reduce postoperative delays.

Giving advice to patients about self-help groups and providing them with the addresses of support agencies can help them to feel less isolated.

It is important to ensure that patients receive adequate nutrition is taken by the patient on a daily basis to maintain their strength and encourage healing. Vitamins C, D and A plus minerals zinc and magnesium, with high protein and calories, will promote wound healing. Referral to a dietician may be required if there are specialized dietary needs, for example those of vegetarians, diabetics, coeliacs or ethnic minorities.

On the day of surgery, the patient should be prepared according to local protocols. *Anti-embolic stockings* should *not* be worn.

PERI-OPERATIVE PROCEDURE

- Urinary catheterization in the anaesthetic room will enhance comfort over the first few postoperative days.
- Haemodynamic status will be monitored and maintained.
- Prophylactic intravenous antibiotics may be given.

Levels of amputation

- *Digital/ray/transmetatarsal amputation.* This is mostly performed for localized ischaemia, which may be due to trauma or diabetic disease.
- *Partial foot.* This is a disarticulation at the level of the tarsometatarsal (Lisfranc disarticulation) or midtarsal joints (Chopart disarticulation). It is performed in the presence of distal vascular disease or trauma when bypass surgery is contraindicated.
- *Syme's amputation.* This is a talotibial disarticulation which preserves the heel pad.
- *Transtibial amputation.* The two forms of amputation at this level are the long posterior-based myocutaneous flap (Burgess) or the skew flap (Robinson). The optimal length for the stump is 14–15 cm, as this will permit good results in fitting a functional modern prosthesis. Measurements are taken from the tibial plateau (Fig. 10.3).
- *Through-knee amputation.* The techniques used are disarticulation of the joints and Gritti-Stokes amputation. Disarticulation does not involve the cutting of muscle or bone, and allows early weight-bearing and limb-fitting. Rotational stability is produced by preserving the patella. The technique cannot be used in the presence of osteoarthritis of the knee. The Gritti-Stokes technique involves excision of the articular surfaces of the patella and femur. The raw surfaces are placed together, which allows them to fuse.
- *Transfemoral amputation.* This is the most common site for amputation. The femur is divided and rounded off to reduce the risk of it penetrating the soft tissues at a later date. A muscle flap is fashioned from the quadriceps and hamstring muscles to form a pad at the stump end. It is important that, during surgery, the surgeon leaves a sufficient length of stump to enable the prosthetist to cast a socket that will accommodate this securely. If the stump is too long, the

Fig. 10.3 A bilateral amputee who has undergone above- and below-knee muscle flap amputations.

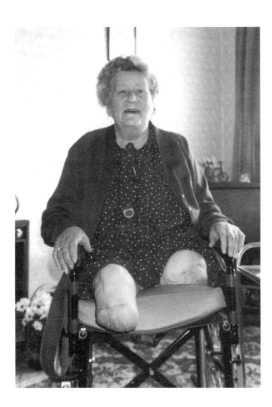

prosthetic knee joint will protrude beyond the other leg, which will be aesthetically and functionally unacceptable.

• *Hip and hindquarter amputation.* This is indicated where there is severe aorto-iliac ischaemia, trauma, severe bone infection or tumours.

• *Upper limb amputations.* These are less frequent, but may be indicated following a critical ischaemic episode due to thromboembolism, vasospastic disorder or trauma. Where the limb has become an encumbrance owing to denervation of the brachial plexus, the amputation is performed across the humerus with fusion of the shoulder joint.

POSTOPERATIVE CONSIDERATIONS

Continual monitoring of haemodynamics, oxygen saturation, respiration and temperature will be required until the patient is fully conscious. These observations can be scaled down in accordance with the stability of the patient's postoperative condition.

Oxygen as prescribed may be given after the operation to assist recovery from the anaesthetic. Oximetry will ascertain whether or not adequate saturation is being achieved.

Ongoing attention to pressure relief will need to be maintained. The use of the monkey pole should be encouraged to reduce the risk of pressure sores caused by friction and sustained interface pressure between the skin and the mattresses.

Routine catheterization will reduce the need for the patient to get out of bed to pass urine, so decreasing the risk of discomfort in the early postoperative days. It will also allow for accurate evaluation of the patient's state of hydration. To reduce the risk of infection, catheters are removed at the earliest possible time, depending on the patient's mobility.

Adequate nutrition and hydration need to be maintained. The diet should be rich in essential nutrients in order to promote wound healing, and should be tailored to any special needs, for example diabetic requirement. Supplementation of dietary intake with highly nutritious formula drinks may help to boost nutritional intake to meet the heavy demands on the patient's stores in the early postoperative phase.

For the amputee who will be mobilizing either on a prosthesis or from a wheelchair, additional calorie intake must be allowed for (Table 10.1) (Osbourne 1992).

Blood will be screened postoperatively for full blood count and urea and electrolytes, and the appropriate measures taken if there is any abnormal blood chemistry or count. Any intravenous cannula is normally removed once prescribed intravenous antibiotics have been discontinued.

The wound requires close observation for haemorrhage and careful dressing techniques to reduce the risk of infection.

A *Redivac drain* is normally left in place for at least 24 hours and the level of exudate should be recorded daily.

The stump dressing is usually not removed for the first 3 days. After this the wound may require dressing on a regular basis until a bandage is no longer required. It is important not to constrict blood flow to the stump or damage delicate tissues through the inappropriate use of tape; therefore a light gauze, retention stump bandage or Tubifast is often used to hold any necessary dressings in place. Skin closures may be removed between the 14th and 17th day after surgery, depending on how quickly the skin heals.

When the incision line is secure, it is useful for patients to wear a '*Juzo stump sock*', which provides shaped light compression. This helps to reduce oedema and to mould the stump to a shape that will comfortably fit into a prosthesis, should one be used.

Ongoing pain relief has to be maintained in a bid to reduce the intensity of phantom sensation and pain. Encouraging the patient to look at the stump and hold the end of it will help the brain to make necessary accommodation to the loss of the limb. All pre-operative pain-control interventions can be maintained, but postoperatively the need for opiates should be considerably reduced.

> A Juzo stump sock:
>
> - reduces oedema
> - moulds the stump to fit a prosthesis
> - is only used when the suture line is secure.

Sleep

Having freedom from pain can improve an amputee's sleep, strength and quality of life, so generating more enthusiasm to take up new hobbies which restore a sense of gratification and self-actualization. This will promote positive acceptance of an amputation.

Mobilization

From the first postoperative day, providing there are no coexisting complications, amputees should be encouraged to take up the independent activities required for daily living. It may be enough for them to stay in bed on the first postoperative day and aim to sit out in a chair for a short while on the second day. Depending on their agility, patients may transfer using a Zimmer frame, but only in order to swivel from their bed to the chair. Hopping can put excessive pressures and increased metabolic demands on the remaining limb, and if there is coexisting peripheral vascular disease this is not advisable. Sitting in a chair will help to strengthen an amputee's back, as the altered centre of gravity places extra demands on the muscles of the back to support an upright position. Rolling over in bed and sitting up will also require adjustments in muscle activity and movement.

Lying face down for short periods of the day, providing the patient does not become breathless, will help to strengthen the gluteal muscles and reduce the risk of flexion contractures. Patients who are able to tolerate abduction of the stump and bridging, which entails lifting their buttocks off the bed, will benefit from increased muscle tone in their stump when they mobilize in a prosthesis.

It is more pleasant for patients to be taken out to the toilet than to have to defecate in an open ward. There is no reason why they cannot be lifted onto a commode and wheeled into the bathroom in the early days if they are unable to transfer from their bed to the commode independently.

It is important to remember that a special sling will be required to accommodate the bilateral amputee, who may experience a sense of falling forward owing to the altered centre of gravity.

Hygiene

As soon as the stump incision has knitted together, patients can bath or shower. Careful hygiene will help to reduce the risk of infection. It is essential that patients look after the stump, but looking after any remaining limb is equally important. For those who are diabetic, referral to a diabetic clinic for regular check-ups and advice regarding diet, hygiene and footwear is beneficial.

The following topics should be discussed with the patient:

- skin care and hygiene in general
- care of the stump, observing for any cyanosis, trauma, pressure, protrusion of bone, infection, pain and flexion contractures
- care of the artificial limb, where this is appropriate.

The patient should be taught how to care for the prosthesis once it has been fitted.
The patient should be advised to:

- wipe out the socket of the limb on a daily basis, using a clean damp cloth and mild soap
- wash the silicone sock and inner liners in lukewarm soapy water every day, and dry with a cloth
- wash stump socks and the sock for the remaining foot each night, using a non-perfumed soap. They should be hand washed and not dried in a tumble-drier
- contact the prosthetist immediately if any repairs are required to the prosthesis. The patient and his carers should not attempt to make adjustments or perform repair work themselves
- ensure that the height of new shoes is identical to that of the old, as any change will alter the gait and may cause the patient to fall. If the height is to be changed, adjustments should be made to the settings of the artificial limb prior to wearing the new shoes
- check stumps regularly for redness, blistering, pressure sores or protruding bone and, if there are any signs of this, seek professional help immediately
- wash any remaining foot and stump/s daily, but do not soak them for too long, as this will soften the tissues and allow infection to enter. Skin should be kept moist and supple with a light emollient. Massaging the stump will help to reduce phantom sensation.

Appliances and stump socks

Long-term appliances have become very sophisticated in recent years; they now range from simple stylish suspension prostheses to silicone Iceross prostheses and to prostheses with intelligent knees. Sophisticated feet, which are now available, incorporate energy-absorbing material that creates more dynamic movement in the foot. The prosthesis is chosen to match the needs of the individual (Fig. 10.4).

Over a period of time, the stump will shrink as the oedema lessens and the inactive muscle becomes wasted. To accommodate this, extra stump socks will need to be worn with a prosthesis in order to ensure that the stump fits snugly into the prosthetic socket.

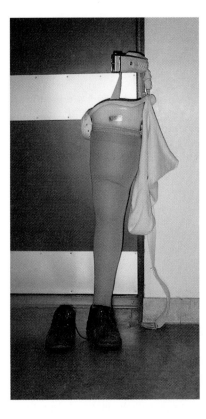

Fig. 10.4 Artificial limbs are dressed to be cosmetically attractive, in accordance with the individual amputee's taste.

REHABILITATION FOLLOWING AN AMPUTATION

Rehabilitation may be defined as re-education following injury or illness that will support people's efforts to maximize their independence.

At the beginning of the rehabilitation phase it is important to work in a collaborative way with the patients and to help them to set attainable goals. Rehabilitation is considered to have failed if the patient continues to focus on the amputation. When preoccupation with this has gone and the person is able to concentrate on other aspects of life, rehabilitation is seen to be successful.

Many professionals will be involved with the patient during the rehabilitation phase and communication is essential to success. The patient is the most important member in the team and should be seen to be making decisions again about his or her own future.

Enhancing self-esteem will boost the process of rehabilitation. Over the forth-coming weeks, the aim is to promote independence in day-to-day activities within the limits of the individual's potential. Wearing day clothes rather than nightwear during the day will promote self-esteem. Patients should be encouraged to share their feelings with their carers: 'A problem shared is a problem halved'. Support and advice should be made available as required. The support of the multidisciplinary team in improving physical skills is also of value in promoting a better quality of life for the amputee.

Emotional rehabilitation

Following amputation the patient will be dealing with emotions which may range from denial and anger to euphoria and overacceptance before appropriate acceptance is possible. Denial can express itself in many ways: for example, emotions may be deflected at carers—others are blamed for the problem. The patient may continue to refuse to accept the disability and try to do as he or she did before. Signs of overacceptance may present as giving in to the disability, or overidentifying with the disability and using this as an excuse for withdrawing from social contacts. The support of a trained counsellor will help the patient to address these emotions, and to move forward and concentrate on the process of physical rehabilitation.

Patients need time to grieve for the loss of a limb and lifestyle. In the eighteenth century, William Cowper stated: 'Grief is itself a medicine'. Apart from the fact that the grieving must be allowed to take its course, in the early postoperative days patients may still be recuperating from the high levels of analgesia and sedation they required before the operation. Both the drugs and the potentially toxic nature of the underlying disease process may have induced some amnesia. The fact that they have lost a limb may seem confusing and unreal. Trying to piece together events leading up to the amputation may stimulate emotions of anger and frustration. Psychological assistance is often needed to help the patient to understand why amputation was necessary and to come to terms with this.

All patients undergoing amputation should be encouraged to take one day at a time. Gaining confidence in their altered lifestyle is a lengthy process. It often helps if they can set themselves a long-term *realistic goal*, which may be something as simple as being able to go back to their lunch club, or to revisit the hairdresser or library on a weekly basis. They may have a forthcoming family event that they can aim to attend, even if they do so in a wheelchair. It is important that they realize that they are respected and loved for the people they are, and not for their limbs. Individuals have many positive attributes to contribute to society and their families. Positively highlighting the value of their contributions will raise self-esteem and strengthen the will to recover.

Wherever possible, as professionals working within the multidisciplinary team, we aim to reduce the impact that amputation will have on patients' lives. We should endeavour to achieve this by helping them to adapt by using new skills, and by offering advice on any beneficial changes that can be made to their environment, or on equipment available that will allow maximum independence.

Physiotherapy

Enabling the patient to move from bed to chair, chair to chair and chair to toilet will increase independence. The use of a slide board will be demonstrated, and support will be given until self-sufficiency is achieved. Exercises to strengthen arms—for example, throwing a ball and extending a rubber band—will help to attain this. Ending the stump to the side promotes flexion in the joints. If possible, the physiotherapist will show patients how to stand on one leg and take their weight when transferring from one seat to another. Sitting in a chair helps to strengthen the patient's back as he learns to adjust the position of his centre of gravity to cope with the loss of the lower limbs. This can be tiring in the early stages and needs to be balanced with periods of rest. Simple manoeuvres such as turning over and sitting up from supine will need practice in order to accommodate the body's new centre of gravity.

After the operation it is important to take the patient to the gym as soon as possible so that rehabilitation can begin; this will generate a positive outlook.

It is important to assess patients as soon as possible to establish whether or not they will be able to manage to mobilize safely on an artificial limb. To do so requires strength, free joint mobility and an efficient cardiopulmonary system. Therefore patients who are blind or who experience paraesthesiae, arthritis or cardiac or pulmonary insufficiency will not be immediately identifiable as suitable candidates for a prosthesis. It is important to establish exactly what rehabilitation the patient would like, and to weigh this against the experience of the professionals involved in rehabilitation, so that the individual's potential can be fully realized within his or her recognized limitations.

For those patients who are aiming to mobilize independently in a wheelchair, ongoing support will be given in training them to transfer from and to the wheelchair, on and off the toilet, to and from the bed, in and out of the bath, in and out of a car, and on and off the floor in case they fall, and to stand independently. Patients who mobilize using a prosthesis will also be trained to manage different floor surfaces, both inside and outside. Walking up and down stairs can pose quite a challenge, but for the strong, healthy agile patient this skill should be attainable.

The level of comprehension and motivation that patients demonstrate will influence their rate of progress, as will their courage and trust in those supporting them.

Before a prosthesis is fitted, early mobility aids (EMA) can be used to assess patients' longer-term ability to cope with an artificial limb. Some of the better-known models are the pneumatic post-amputation mobility aid (Fig. 10.5), Femurett and Tulip. Whichever EMA is used, the aim will be to maintain balance and spatial awareness while wearing a prosthesis to develop muscle control and hip extension in the stance phase of the gait cycle, and to move independently between parallel bars.

Occupational therapy (OT)

Once the surgery has been completed and the patient is feeling stronger, he or she may be taken to the OT department for everyday activity assessment. A date will be set for a home visit to evaluate the ability of the patient to cope at home, and this information will be of value when planning discharge.

Referral to a rehabilitation centre

Where appropriate, patients will be given an appointment with the artificial limb centre, where they will be assessed and assisted in their rehabilitation. Even patients who are not receiving either a cosmetic prosthesis or an artificial limb may still require assistance from a rehabilitation centre in manoeuvring a wheelchair over different surfaces or in learning transfer skills. If necessary, arrangements can be made for follow-up physiotherapy on an outpatient basis until patients have achieved as much physical independence as possible.

DISCHARGE FROM HOSPITAL

Patients will only be discharged when they are ready to cope back in the community. The hospital staff will ensure that all necessary supports have been organized.

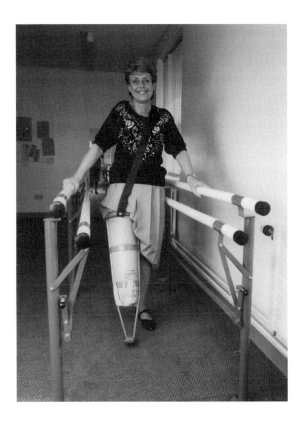

Fig. 10.5 Walking at the earliest possible time with an early walking aid, such as a PPAM aid, between parallel bars will help to promote self-confidence and self-esteem. (Reproduced with kind permission from Vessa Ltd.)

In line with the Community Care Act, this will require a multi-agency assessment (MAA). The patient is now moving from the security of a protected environment to the real world, where he or she will have to face other members of society and learn to get around using a new form of mobility. It is not easy for everyone to face the world again and adapt to their new body image. Ongoing counselling and physiotherapy support may be required for many months until a full adjustment has been made.

Any medicines should be ordered on the day before discharge, so that there is no delay once the patient is ready to leave the hospital. A letter will be sent to the patient's general practitioner (GP), so enabling any further supplies to be prescribed as needed. It is important that patients know that they should contact their doctor in good time for renewals, as it is normal for hospitals to provide only a few days' supply on discharge.

If the skin closures are still in place when the patient is discharged, arrangements will need to be made for their removal. This is usually with the district nurse. However, it is uncommon for patients to leave a clinical setting at such an early stage: most consultants will wish to ensure that the wound has healed together before transferring patients from an acute surgical ward to a community hospital, a nursing home or their own home for convalescence.

Once discharged from hospital, the provision of a rehabilitation programme will continue. Arrangements will need to be made with the agencies described above to ensure that all relevant supports are safely in place.

• *Returning to work.* If this is applicable, patients may return to work as soon as they feel able after checking the most appropriate timing for this with their consultant or GP and employer. However, they may require some retraining, and the support of the local placing, assessment and counselling teams (PACT), who offer a comprehensive service to help people return to work, will be beneficial.

• *Working at home.* There is no restriction on physical activity at home. Patients need to be encouraged to be as active as possible.

• *Exercise.* Continuing the exercises taught in hospital will promote independent mobility. It is important for amputees to keep as fit as possible. Local swimming baths are very accommodating, and swimming is a good exercise often enjoyed by people who have had an amputation.

• *Diet.* Unless there is some other underlying medical condition, there is no restriction on diet. However, one should always bear in mind the benefits of a healthy diet.

• *Smoking.* If the patient stopped smoking before the operation, encouragement not to start again may help patients keep to this, so reducing the risk of further peripheral vascular disease, coronary and respiratory disease.

• *Alcohol.* In order to maintain a healthy lifestyle, patients should not exceed the recommended daily limit.

• *Bathing.* Before discharge, the occupational therapist will have assessed the home situation and the patients' ability in this activity. There is no restriction on bathing, provided that patients feel able to cope with the arrangements. Home alterations can be organized by social services to meet individual needs: examples are wheel-in shower units, ramps to replace steps, stair or through-ceiling lifts and the lowering of units to accommodate wheelchairs.

• *Home support.* This should be in place before the patient goes home, and a period of convalescence at a community hospital may be required in order to achieve this, as well as allowing the patient to regain the ability to cope independently.

• *Sexual activities.* Patients can resume a normal sex life as soon as they feel happy about doing so.

• *Driving.* If appropriate, arrangements can be made to adapt cars to the satisfaction of the DVLA, to enable patients to continue to drive. If they are under 65, they may be entitled to a mobility allowance, so enabling them to adapt their car and to ensure that they are able to carry a wheelchair if needed. Advice can be obtained from the Disabled Driver Association. Patients will need to inform the DVLA of their changed situation. Their doctors will tell them when they are able to drive again. Applications for disability badges ('orange badges') may be obtained from social services.

• *Constant Care Line.* This is a telephone-based service which gives patients constant contact with an emergency help line. A cordless remote control can be worn as a pendant or clipped onto clothing. Should the patient not be within reach of the telephone and need instant help in an emergency, simply pressing the remote control button will establish voice-to-voice contact with the service. A referral by the service can then be made to close relatives or to the patient's general practitioner.

SAMPLE CLINICAL GUIDELINES FOR THE CARE OF PATIENTS UNDERGOING AMPUTATION

Amputee check list

Prior to attendance at rehabilitation centre for limb fitting		
Action	**Date**	**Signature**

Pre-operative
- *Pressure risk assessment* and necessary aids are in place pre-operatively.
- *A monkey pole* is in place pre-operatively.
- *Height and weight* have been recorded.

Postoperative
- *Urinary catheter bag* tubing is hung on the opposite side to the newly formed stump.
- *Chairs and commodes* are placed on the opposite side of the bed to that which has just undergone amputation.
- *Dressings* are held in place using a Tubifast bandage only.
- *No tape* is applied to the stump (yellow line Tubifast for AKA, blue line for BKA).

Pain control
- The patient is made aware of phantom sensation and knows he or she should think consciously about not stepping onto a phantom limb.
- The patient has been told to request analgesia if required.
- Massage to reduce phantom sensation has been demonstrated.

Movement
- For BKA elevation of stump, to be level with the hips, keeping the knee straight, has been requested of the patient.
- AKA have been requested to hold the stump vertically when standing and to keep it flat against the bed and not elevated on pillows.
- The patient is able to transfer from bed to chair using a Zimmer frame and *does not hop*.
- Dynamic exercises have been demonstrated by the physiotherapist and are being implemented by the patient.

The patient has been referred to:
- the vascular nurse practitioner
- the occupational therapist
- the rehabilitation centre
- the physiotherapist.

A wheelchair request has been sent off with a request for tyre pump, pressure relief devices, stump boards where applicable, weight and height of patient, level of amputation, status of amputee (bilateral or unilateral).

The patient has been informed that he/she will *attend the gym* at the hospital and how frequently.

Cont'd

Amputee check list cont'd

Action	Date	Signature

If the patient is likely to benefit from a prosthesis, he/she is being encouraged to use the PPAM aid by the 7th–10th day to help reduce oedema in the stump and phantom limb sensation.

The patient is able to discuss realistic goals and desires rehabilitation.

The patient has been given advice about *driving and financial benefits.*

A referral to social services has been made if appropriate to address the need for home care, meals on wheels.

A date for a *home visit* has been set with the *occupational therapist.*

The patient is *aware of the process of rehabilitation* in agreement with the consultant.

The patient has been measured for a *Juzo stocking* to shape the stump.

On referral for rehabilitation the centre has been made aware of:
- coexisting conditions
- age, gender, GP's telephone number, name of consultant
- status of amputation (AKA, BKA, Syme's, bilateral, unilateral), name of ward they are currently on or will be sent to, home address
- the presence of MRSA (this will not delay/prohibit referral); a separate ambulance has been booked for anyone with generalized MRSA
- medication required whilst at the centre
- continence status.

On the day of attendance at the centre the patient should take with him/her:
- the physiotherapist's, occupational therapist's and nursing reports
- medical notes and prescription chart
- any medication, including analgesia, required for that day
- shoes and socks
- a pair of shorts or a short skirt (not long trousers).

Prior to attending, patients should be encouraged to continue to take any *diuretics* to reduce the risk of oedema of the stump. They have been told to ask *anyone* if they wish to use the toilet as they will be at the centre for most of the day.

They are aware that they will meet the full multidisciplinary team at the centre, including the doctor, nurse, occupational therapist, physio, counsellor, and prosthetist if appropriate.

Hygiene When patients have a prosthesis, they are aware of the need to wash stump socks and the inside of the prosthesis regularly.

Relatives are aware of supports which are available to them.

REFERENCES

Astill G 1993 The phantom phenomena—what's new? Step Forward (Journal for the
    Limbless Association) 30: 7–8
Norgren L 1990 Definition, incidence and epidemiology. In: Dormandy J A, Stock G (eds)
    Critical limb ischaemia: its pathophysiology and management. Springer-Verlag, Berlin
Sedgwick E M 1993 Phantom limbs. Step Forward (Journal for the Limbless Association) 25:
    1–2

FURTHER READING

American Academy of Orthopaedic Surgeons 1991 Atlas for amputation surgery and
    prosthetics, 2nd edn.
Amputee Rehabilitation Society 1992 A report by the working party. Royal College of
    Physicians, London
Barsby P, Lumley J S P 1987 Checklist for the management of the lower limb amputee.
    Surgery 1(41): 985–986
Dormandy J A, Ray S A 1994 The fate of amputees. Vascular Medicine Review 5: 331–346
Dormandy J A, Thomas P R S 1988 What is the natural history of a critically ischaemic
    patient with and without his leg? In: Greenhalgh R M, Jamison C W, Nicolaides A N
    (eds) Limb salvage and amputation for vascular disease. Saunders, Philadelphia
Engstrom B, Van de Van C 1985 Physiotherapy for amputees—the Roehampton approach.
    Churchill Livingstone, Edinburgh
Hallett J W Jr, Brewster D C, Clement Darling R Jr 1995 Handbook of patient care in vascular
    surgery, 3rd edn. Little, Brown, Boston
Ham R O, Thornberry D J, Regan J F et al 1986 The management of the lower limb amputee
    in England and Wales today. Physiotherapy Practice 2: 94–100
Humm J 1973 Rehabilitation of the lower limb amputee, 3rd edn. Baillière Tindall, London
Lein S 1992 How are physiotherapists using the vessa pneumatic post-amputation mobility
    aid? Physiotherapy 78(5): 318–322
Murdoch G, Donovan J (eds) 1988 Amputation surgery and lower limb prosthetics.
    Blackwell, Oxford
Robinson K P, Hoile R, Coddington T 1982 Skew flap myoplastic below knee amputation: a
    preliminary report. British Journal of Surgery 69: 554–557
Vitali M, Robinson K P, Andrews B G, Harris E E, Readhead R 1986 Amputations and
    prostheses, 2nd edn. Baillière Tindall, London

Caring for the patient undergoing abdominal aortic aneurysm repair

This chapter will address the needs of patients undergoing reconstruction surgery for an abdominal aortic aneurysm (AAA).

The incidence of aortic aneurysm is highest in Western males over the age of 65, especially where there is a history of smoking, high stress, raised blood cholesterol levels and familial presentation. It is thought that females may be given some protection from circulating levels of oestrogen. Above the age of 80, the incidence among males and females evens out.

Patients presenting with an abdominal aortic aneurysm, as seen in Figure 11.1, may be referred by their general practitioner for vascular surgery, come through the accident and emergency department, be referred by urologists or be picked up from screening programmes for males over the age of 65 (the latter will possibly be advocated by the as yet unpublished Chichester Study).

Screening by ultrasound in the over-65 age group is now in progress in many centres in the UK, often in GPs' surgeries. In some centres, patients with aneurysms measuring between 2.5 and 5 cm are invited for repeat screening every 9 months. Those with aneurysms of over 5 cm diameter are offered conventional surgery if their general physical condition permits. Some centres are now offering surgery at an earlier stage, when endovascular surgery is now becoming an option.

Where surgery is elective, the mortality rate is between 5 and 8%. This varies from centre to centre. The presentation of the patient and variations in coexisting disease will contribute to these anomalies. For example, between 50–70% of patients presenting will also have heart disease and 40–60% may well have experienced a previous myocardial infarction. Other coexisting conditions are diabetes,

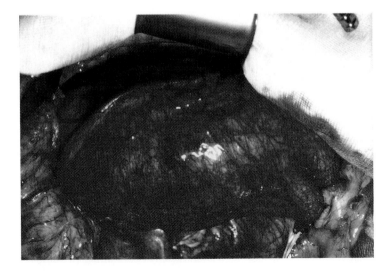

Fig. 11.1 A large aortic aneurysm.

hypertension, respiratory disorders and renal failure due to generalized micro- or macrovascular disease.

Contraindications for AAA repair are:

- extreme age
- concurrent malignancy with a poor prognosis
- unrecordable blood pressure, or a neurologically unresponsive patient.

Where the patient is considered to be generally unfit for anaesthesia but carries a high risk of rupture and morbidity, he may prefer to take the chance of having surgery if it will save his life, in which case it is acceptable to offer him this opportunity. The balance has to be drawn between being realistic and offering a chance of survival.

In some cases the position and size of the proximal neck of the aneurysm is such that will not allow sufficient space to anastomose a graft. Involvement of the renal arteries in the aneurysm will increase the technical complexity of the procedure and may be a relative contraindication.

Complications arising from AAA surgery are:

- myocardial infarction, which can occur as late as the 3rd postoperative day, and carries the highest risk of mortality
- congestive cardiac failure
- pulmonary embolus
- chest infection
- renal failure
- infarcted bowel
- paralytic ileus
- cerebrovascular accident
- ischaemic lower limbs
- deep vein thrombosis
- impotence
- graft failure.

INVESTIGATIONS NEEDED BEFORE A DECISION IS MADE TO OFFER SURGERY

A full blood count, urea and electrolytes, creatinine clearance and blood lipids are essential, as are a chest X-ray, lung function tests and an ECG. Thirty per cent of patients with no previous history of a myocardial infarction will present with changes in their ECG following an exercise test. An echogram of the heart is considered by some to be the most effective way of establishing whether the patient has an increased risk of myocardial infarction postoperatively. Cardiac catheterization may be required, or a thallium study to demonstrate the ability of the heart to cope under stress. As coronary angiogram can increase the risk of myocardial infarction, it tends to be reserved for times when a decision to operate on a high-risk patient hangs in the balance. It is common to perform an ultrasound scan of the aneurysm and/or a CT scan. Where there is access to magnetic resonance imaging, a clearer view of the situation can be obtained.

Angiography (arteriogram) may be required to establish the position of the aneurysm.

As a result of developments in radiological studies, it is becoming possible to use a spiral scanner to perform multiseeded, 3D CT angiography which will allow different structures within and around the aneurysm to be accurately defined and measured, so permitting more precise diagnosis and surgery, especially regarding the insertion of stents during endovascular surgery.

PATIENT PREPARATION FOR SURGERY

Learning that major surgical intervention is being suggested can be frightening and confusing for patients. Emotional, physical and educational support may help to reduce patients' anxiety and enable them to become involved and pro-active in their preparation for surgery and recovery.

Health promotion

It is important that the patient is as fit as possible prior to admission. As outlined in Chapter 3, health promotion before and after the operation will enhance the patient's quality of life and reduce the risk of complications. Lifestyle issues may be addressed in the pre-operative waiting period, so reducing risk factors. The growth rate of small aneurysms over 3 years was found to be lower in patients who stopped smoking from the outset (MacSweeney et al 1994).

PRE-OPERATIVE CARE

The patient is usually admitted on the day before surgery.

It is important that there is sufficient planning, so that the appropriate nursing skill mix is available to provide adequate care for a patient undergoing major aortic reconstruction surgery.

Once the patient's needs in relation to day-to-day activities and pressure relief have been identified, and a full nursing assessment has been carried out, the object of care will be to ensure that predetermined goals have been achieved by the time the patient is discharged.

Admission to the ward prior to surgery will allow patients time for physical and psychological adjustment, as they become familiar with the new environment and with members of the multidisciplinary team. If patients so wish, it may also be appropriate for them to visit the clinical area in which they will be placed immediately after the operation—for example, a high-dependency or intensive care unit.

A full nursing and medical history will need to be given to all members of the care team and documented accurately. Any special needs or allergies should be taken into consideration and any risk factors identified.

Anaesthesia

The anaesthetist will assess the cardiorespiratory status prior to anaesthesia and discuss postoperative management of pain with the patient. It has been established that the level of pain increases the higher the surgical incision goes up the abdominal wall. Ineffective pain control will lead to poor respiratory action of the chest wall, resulting in pooling of secretions and guarding, which will inhibit the patient's movements while increasing the risk of chest infection. Pain stimulates the sympathetic nervous system, giving rise to increased cardiac stress.

Epidural pain relief is often the mode chosen, and the drugs of choice are bupivacaine and diamorphine. An anti-emetic may need to be included to reduce nausea.

Respiratory depression is a side-effect of morphine-based drugs and this may not show until as late as 24 hours after the beginning of the infusion. When monitoring, it is not enough to observe only the rate of respiration, as the rate does not reflect the level of sedation that will need to be established to ensure appropriate control. Should the epidural be found to be ineffective postoperatively, it may be that it has become dislodged from its site. Care of the epidural site to reduce the risk of infection entering and the leakage of CSF will need to be maintained. Should the epidural fail, it is wiser to remove the catheter and use a patient-controlled analgesic system instead, or intramuscular injections at regular intervals as prescribed.

The physiotherapist should assess patients, informing them sensitively as to possible complications and stressing the importance of passive leg exercises to reduce the risk of deep vein thrombosis postoperatively. Breathing exercises may reduce the risk of chest infections.

Some of the investigations performed in outpatients may be repeated—for example, blood screening for urea and electrolytes and full blood count. The patient will be cross-matched for blood; 6 units are often requested. The pro-thrombin time may be established and in anticoagulated patients warfarin will be discontinued 24 hours prior to surgery and replaced with heparin. The APTT will need close monitoring to reduce the risk of clotting or haemorrhage.

ECG, echogram and chest X-ray and a CT scan or ultrasound of the aneurysm may also be repeated.

On the day of admission, it is appropriate to start compiling a discharge plan to ensure that all supports are in place when needed.

Useful baseline observations are blood pressure and pulse, ward urinalysis, and ward blood glucose test. Doppler ultrasound to detect the presence of pedal pulses will evaluate perfusion to the lower limbs.

The use of a recognized tool—for example, the Waterlow scale or Norton scale—to assess the risk of pressure sore development will enable nursing staff to provide pressure relief equipment and to intervene to prevent sores from developing either during or after surgery.

The patient's weight and height should be recorded pre-operatively to establish body mass index and to permit the monitoring of weight loss and nutrition postoperatively. The nutritional status of the patient will affect wound healing, and attention needs to be paid to this postoperatively to ensure a good recovery.

Should diabetes coexist with aortic aneurysm, the patient may need sliding scale insulin pre-operatively until blood sugars are stable. Any special dietary needs should be communicated to the dietician and members of the multidisciplinary team.

In some centres an abdominal shave may be requested. Hair is removed from below the nipple to the top of the pubis, incorporating the groins and tops of the legs, as it may be necessary to explore the iliac arteries during surgery. The shave may be performed in surgery or not at all, depending on the surgeon's preferences.

Informed consent to anaesthesia and surgery *must* be obtained.

No diet or fluids should be taken for 6 hours prior to surgery except in an emergency, in which case H_2-receptor blockers, e.g. ranitidine, are given to reduce stomach acidity. This will make it less likely, in the event of vomit being inhaled, that Mendelson's syndrome—i.e. severe spasm of the bronchioles caused by inhalation of acid from the stomach—will occur. Regular essential medication—for example, antihypertensive therapy—should still be given orally both before and after surgery, in spite of the nil-by-mouth order.

Anti-embolic stockings may be requested to reduce the risk of deep vein thrombosis, provided that there is no evidence of arterial insufficiency to the lower limbs.

Finally, a premedication anaesthetic should be dispensed as prescribed.

OPERATIVE TECHNIQUE

During surgery the patient is intubated. Haemodynamics and urine output are closely monitored during anaesthesia, and heparin is used to reduce thrombus formation in the distal vessels.

In elective surgery, the surgeon opens the abdominal wall and locates the aorta by moving the bowel to one side. Clamps are placed above and below the aneurysm to establish a controlled environment before the aneurysmal sac is opened and the exact location and size of the aneurysm explored. Where the iliac arteries are involved, a trouser graft will be required. Should the renal arteries be aneurysmal or at risk of occlusion from the insertion of a graft, consideration will need to be given as to whether or not to continue, given the possibility of an ongoing need for renal dialysis postoperatively.

In a straightforward procedure, the thrombus is scooped out of the aorta prior to the insertion of a graft (made of dacron, a synthetic material) at the proximal end (Fig. 11.2). A sample of the thrombus is sent for culture, as in 15% of cases infection is present and antibiotics will be required to protect the graft from failing.

The dacron graft is carefully measured to ensure that the size is exact, so reducing the risk of kinking or overstretching on insertion, which could lead respectively to occlusion of the graft or leakage from the anastomosis once the graft is under pressure from the blood flow. Caution is used in releasing the proximal clamp to ensure that there is no leakage from the anastomosis. The surgeon repeats the procedure for the distal end before closing the aorta back around the graft.

With the advent of endovascular techniques and the insertion of aortic stents through the femoral artery, accessed through a small incision in the groin (Yusuf et al 1994), it is anticipated that AAA repair will be moving into a new and exciting phase that will provide treatment for patients with far less surgical trauma. At the time of writing, less than 1000 abdominal aortic stents have been inserted—and these have been for small, infrarenal aneurysms—but the progress of this procedure is under the close scrutiny of the medical press. Only time will tell if the use of this developing technique will produce the lasting results that are hoped for.

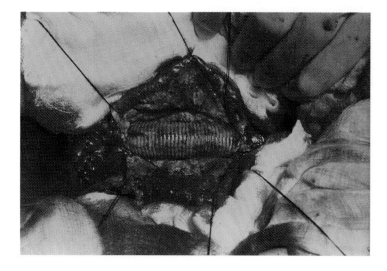

Fig. 11.2 Aortic graft in situ.

Initial postoperative care of AAA patient:

- general intensive care nursing
- monitoring of cardiovascular system
  — arterial and CVP lines
  — oximetry
- monitoring of pulmonary function: possible need for ventilation
- monitoring of renal function
- pain control via epidural infusion
- NG tube + parenteral feeding until bowel functional
- Doppler assessment of pedal pulses
- protection of limbs and pressure points.

POSTOPERATIVE CONSIDERATIONS

After conventional surgery, if the patient is intubated he or she will be nursed in an intensive care unit. Otherwise the patient will usually return to a high-dependency area for the first 48 hours or until stable (Fig. 11.3).

For the first 24–48 hours, the patient's internal environment will be continuously evaluated by the use of monitors, so ensuring a prompt response should there be any destabilization of his condition. Nursing activity will include monitoring cardiopulmonary activity, the state of hydration, renal function, gastrointestinal function, levels of pain, signs of haemorrhage or infection, and perfusion to the lower limbs.

It is important to remember that the aorta is the major trunk from which other major arterial vessels stem. Any intra-operative trauma to these vessels may result in renal failure, bowel infarction or ischaemia of the lower limbs. There is a high risk of myocardial infarction within the first 3 days, and pulmonary embolism is always a postoperative risk.

Ongoing nursing assessment of the patient's needs and potential and actual problems will enable management to be sensitive, responsive and relevant to the situation. This will help to guarantee quality of care in the postoperative phase. Alongside monitoring, adequate attention should be given to meeting the basic needs of the patient in regard to day-to-day activities.

Care of the patient's hygiene, oral care whilst nil by mouth, care of limbs to protect them from being strained or knocked while the patient is semiconscious, communication of positive information to help reduce anxiety and ensure that the patient can relax and sleep will all contribute towards a comfortable postoperative period.

Whilst patients are bed-bound there is a risk of them developing pressure sores, and all precautions should be taken to prevent this.

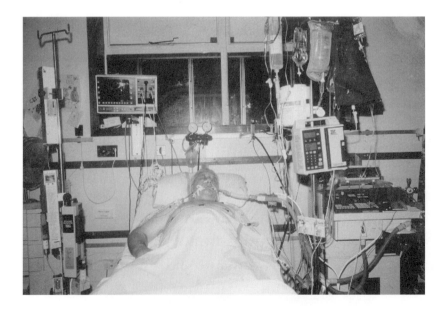

Fig. 11.3 ITU monitoring after aortic aneurysm surgery. (Reproduced with kind permission from Mr Paterson, Goodhope NHS Trust.)

During surgery, it is possible for small emboli to be thrown off, and these may occlude the distal vessels of the leg. Hand-held Doppler ultrasound is useful for assessing accurately the presence of pedal pulses.

An arterial line will be in place from which to establish the vital haemodynamic status. A comparison of postoperative and pre-operative baseline readings will give vital information regarding the individual's central and peripheral arterial perfusion. An intravascular fluid regime will ensure that there is adequate hydration and will balance the serum electrolytes until such time as oral fluids are able to be tolerated.

Intravascular antibiotic cover is usually given for the first 5 days, via the central line, until the patient is able to tolerate light diet. *Pyrexia* may be indicative of infection in the urinary tract, wound, chest or peritoneum.

Oximetry usefully measures the level of arterial oxygen, so that prompt action can be taken should a hypoxic state develop. Intubation may need to be maintained in the early postoperative phase but, after this has been discontinued, the administration of continous pernasal warmed and humidified oxygen for at least 24 hours will reduce the risk of postoperative infarction and hypoxia while the patient is recovering from the anaesthetic. In some centres, overnight oxygen may be prescribed by the anaesthetist for up to 5 postoperative nights to ensure adequate oxygen perfusion to the heart, so reducing cardiac stress and the risk of postoperative myocardial infarction.

By nursing the patient in an upright position and ensuring that deep breathing and chest physiotherapy is maintained, one reduces the risk of bronchial secretions collecting in the lungs and therefore of a chest infection. Holding the abdomen when coughing may aid expectoration, as such support will reduce the associated pain.

Urinary catheterization increases the patient's comfort, manages his or her need to micturate and allows hourly measurement of output, which should be at least 30 ml/h. Where this is found to be low, it may be due either to a drop in blood pressure caused by operative shock, or to haemorrhage, poor pain control or dehydration. Clinical assessment of contributing factors will determine the condition of the patient; for example, the CVP will be recorded to determine the fluid load on the heart.

A low CVP reading and low urine output may indicate reduced blood volume due to either haemorrhage or dehydration. Fluid will be required to improve this situation. Should the CVP be high, the urine output may also be increased, though it is not known why this should be. Reduction of CVP with antihypertensive drugs such as diuretics may establish homoeostasis. A bounding jugular venous pulse may indicate right ventricular failure.

A low urine output in the presence of a normal or high CVP may indicate renal shutdown after the temporary clamping of the renal arteries in theatre. The treatment is i.v. infusion of dopamine. Renal shutdown may be indicative of an acute thrombotic episode or hypotension due to haemorrhage, either of which can lead to renal failure.

Where the urine output does not respond to clinical intervention, renal failure due to occlusion of the renal artery may be suspected. A significantly raised urea and creatinine is indicative of this.

Should the patient be haemorrhaging, there may be evident signs of bleeding, tachycardia, hypotension or distension of the abdomen.

Postoperative blood screening for blood gases, full blood count, Hb, urea and electrolytes, creatinine clearance and ESR will provide useful information regarding postoperative management. The measurement of cardiac enzymes on the third postoperative day will help to establish whether there has been a myocardial infarction. However, it is possible that the creatine phosphokinase (CPK) will be raised anyway, owing to the surgical trauma caused to muscle tissue, and so it is important to ensure that specific cardiac enzymes are requested—i.e. lactate dehydrogenase (LDH) and creatine kinase myocardial band (CKMB).

Analgesia may be given via an epidural catheter. It is important to protect the back and epidural site from trauma. One needs to watch for leakage of CSF and report immediately to the medical team and anaesthetist any such leakage, as well as excessive patient discomfort, pyrexia, change in haemodynamic status, numbness or paralysis in lower limbs, or trauma at the site of the epidural. A protocol is implemented for the care of the patient undergoing continuous epidural infusion of analgesic and anti-emetic drugs.

It is not uncommon for mild damage to occur in the inferior mesenteric artery, owing to either arterial disease or surgical trauma. This will possibly lead to mild ischaemia of the distal colon and lead to a bout of diarrhoea, which tends to be temporary. However, should damage to the superior mesenteric artery arise, full-thickness necrosis of the small intestine may be experienced, leading to peritonitis and death.

Mesenteric ischaemia may be identified by poor bowel sounds, abdominal pain (which may be severe), nausea irrespective of the nasogastric tube, pyrexia and generalized changes in the haemodynamics, with raised volume and acidity of the gastric juices retrieved by the nasogastric tube.

A straight abdominal X-ray, erect and supine if possible, will help to establish whether or not there is a paralytic ileus stimulated by handling of the bowel or ischaemia due to infarction of the mesenteric artery.

After operative handling of the bowel, it takes a few days for effective peristalsis to return. A nasogastric tube will help to reduce any build-up of secretions in the gut. The volume of such secretions requires monitoring. As bowel sounds return, oral fluid intake can be gradually introduced and increased.

Intravenous fluids must be continued until the patient is capable of taking a light diet. It is not unusual for the appetite at first to be small.

A diet rich in protein, vitamins A, C and D, and minerals such as zinc and magnesium will aid wound healing.

The wound will have been closed according to local preference, and the theatre dressing will be removed in 1–3 days, again depending on consultant preference. Any blood or exudate which strikes through this is noted. If the haemorrhage cannot be brought under control, medical help should be called immediately. A Redivac drain may be in place to reduce the risk of haematoma by the aneurysmal sac. This needs to be removed once the level of exudate has reduced significantly.

Doppler assessment of pedal pulses should be compared with the pre-operative assessment.

Returning to the ward

When the patient's condition has become less critical and cardio/pulmonary stabilty is achieved, he or she may return to the ward. At this point the ward nurses record the patient's vital signs; the monitoring and recording is repeated every 2–4 hours for the next 48 hours or for as long as it takes to show that stability has been maintained for 24 hours and beyond. The frequency of monitoring can then be reduced over the following week, depending on the individual situation.

Fluid and dietary intake

Depending on local policy, the patient may have to remain nil by mouth until bowel sounds can be heard. Oral fluids are then introduced gradually, commencing with 30 ml/h, and progressing to 60, 90, then 120 ml of free fluids. At other centres, the consultant will request that the patient drink from day one, as he or she feels able. Any fluids not absorbed will be drained away through the the nasogastric tube. Regular mouth care is required until the patient can care for himself and take a normal diet. The nasogastric tube will be spigoted off once the patient can tolerate at least 60 ml/h. If there is no nausea or vomiting and fluids continue to be tolerated, the nasogastric tube will be removed on the instructions of the medical team. The patient then takes a light diet, which will be designed to take account of any special needs.

The central line is removed when it is no longer needed for CVP monitoring or as a route for hydration or antibiotics. One should ensure that the tip of the catheter is present on removal, and send this tip to microbiology for culture and sensitivity.

Mobility

The patient is mobilized from bed to chair on the second or third postoperative day. The level of mobility is increased each day, as tolerated. Free mobility should be achieved by the fifth postoperative day.

A monkey pole over the bed may aid independent movement while the patient is in bed. Nursing in an upright position aids respiratory function as well as encouraging the patient to expectorate any phlegm. Any green phlegm should be sent for culture and sensitivity and antibiotics should be administered as prescribed.

Reducing the risk of thrombosis

Subcutaneous anti-embolic drug therapy should be administered as prescribed. It is necessary to encourage passive leg exercises to reduce the risk of DVT and to tell patients not to cross their legs. Continued use of anti-embolic stockings is routine only if ABPI remains above 0.8 and no contraindication presents. Washing and checking the patient's legs daily will allow staff to monitor blood flow closely, ensuring that no ischaemic damage to the tissues or silent deep vein thrombosis has occurred.

Scrotal oedema

In the first postoperative days, generalized oedema of the lower limbs may involve the scrotum. The use of ice packs may help to alleviate discomfort.

Wound management

The wound drain is removed after 24–48 hours or when exudate subsides, on the instructions of the medical team. The theatre dressing is taken off on the third day. Skin closures are removed around the 14th–17th postoperative day; the community nurse can do this if the patient has been discharged.

Preparations for discharge

It is important that planning for discharge is begun on the day of admission, to avoid subsequent delays.

Community care is organized as required for individual patients. Drugs to take home may include aspirin, for which a repeat prescription will be required from the patient's GP.

No driving will be allowed until this is deemed safe by the consultant or GP, probably after the postoperative assessment at the outpatient clinic.

The patient should not carry anything heavier than a dinner tray for at least 4 weeks, but should take a brisk walk each day, if possible, and build up exercise tolerance gently, without overstretching the abdominal muscles in the first 6 weeks. It is important to achieve the right balance between rest and gentle exercise.

Impotence after AAA repair:

- Discuss risk pre-operatively with patient
- Refer to erectile dysfunction specialist if necessary.

Sexuality

During the operation, trauma to the sacral plexus may interfere with the action of the parasympathetic system, resulting in impotence postoperatively. This can cause distress to the patient. Should this occur, patients can be referred to an erectile dysfunction specialist, so that supportive care can be given. The patient should be given the opportunity to discuss any concerns regarding sexuality.

Lifestyle

Finally, one should advise the patient about the best way of achieving a healthy lifestyle that will reduce the risk of arterial disease developing further.

SAMPLE CLINICAL GUIDELINES FOR THE CARE OF PATIENTS UNDERGOING ELECTIVE ABDOMINAL AORTIC ANEURYSM SURGERY

Check list

	Date	Signature
Outpatients Males over the age of 60, screened for AAA at GP surgeries. Aneurysms > 2.5—repeat screens every 6 months until 5 cm. > 5 cm—surgery considered with patient following further investigation and discussion re need for surgery and associated risk factors.		
Investigations Admitted from waiting list unless emergency. Usually over the age of 60. Often with multisegmental disease. Microvascular disease may be present in diabetics or patients with rheumatoid arthritis.		
• Investigations performed pre decision to operation.		
Known from ultrasound scan to have an AAA of > 5 cm—Hb, FBC, lipids, urea and electrolytes, Creatinine, CXR, ECG, thallium and CT scan. Coagulation screen. Echocardiogram. Position of AAA is noted and size of the posterior neck of the aneurysm is noted, to ascertain there is sufficient to allow for anastomosis of the graft.		
• Providing there are no contraindications for surgery, e.g. cardiopulmonary complications, advanced carcinoma in the terminal stages, involvement of the renal arteries or a poor short length at the proximal neck to the aneurysm which would make anastomosis difficult, the patient is offered surgery.		
• Patient information and support to reduce anxieties regarding pending surgery and to ensure adequate understanding, so promoting active involvement of the patient in their preparation for surgery. Lifestyle issues, and their active involvement in their anticipated recovery from surgery are addressed to reduce the risk factors associated with vascular disease.		
• Waiting list for AAA repair admission.		
• Admitted to hospital on the day prior to surgery.		
Admitted to the ward Welcome patient and orientate them to surroundings, staff and routine. Routine medical, anaesthetic and nursing assessments including discharge assessment of needs.		

Cont'd

Check list cont'd

	Date	Signature

- Nursing baseline observations of haemodynamic status. Doppler assessment to identify any coexisting ischaemia in lower limbs.
- Pressure risk assessment. Implementation of nursing care to reduce risk of pressure sore development and acquisition of pressure relief equipment as/if needed.
- Weigh patient and establish their body mass index. Alert dietician to any special dietary needs.
- If diabetic—ward test for blood sugar and urinalysis for glucose and ketones. Alert medical staff to any abnormal results. Sliding scale insulin as/if necessary pre- and postoperatively until able to take normal diet and blood sugars become stable within normal limits.
- Clinical investigations need to be repeated 1-2 weeks prior to surgery if fit. If not fit, or presence of renal problems, or anticoagulated using warfarin, investigations are repeated the day before surgery.
  — Chest X-ray
  — ECG, echocardiogram
  — Blood screen—as above and cross-match for 6 units of blood

Ensure ITU or high-dependency bed is available depending on patient's assessed needs postoperatively.

Consent

- Abdominal shave 24 hours pre-operatively—nipple to top of pubis and groins to mid thigh as requested by Medical Team.
- Offer mild enema if prescribed or laxative.
- Reduce anxiety through patient information and emotional support.
- Physiotherapy assessment and information given regarding post-operative intervention to reduce risk of DVT and chest infection.
- Visit high-dependency unit pre-operatively to meet staff and become familiar with environment if patient desires to do so.
- Nil by mouth for 6 hours pre-operatively. Ensure any antihypertensive medication is given orally even when otherwise nil by mouth, both pre- and postoperatively.
- Pre-med if prescribed.

Peri-operatively

- Monitor haemodynamic status.
- Intra-operative heparin to reduce thrombus formation in graft.
- Continued relief of pressure to reduce risk of sores developing interoperatively.

Postoperatively

- Continued pressure relief to reduce risk of pressure sore development.
- Transferred to a high-dependency unit until condition has stabilized (usually 24–48 hours).
- If intubated—transferred to ITU.

Cont'd

Check list cont'd

	Date	Signature

Report to medical staff and anaesthetists any abnormal recordings found in continual monitoring of:

- ECG, BP, pulse (immediately report to medical staff — pulse less then 40, BP < 100/50 > > 190/100).
- Temperature, respiration.
- CVP.
- O2 saturation — if not intubated — nasal O2 as prescribed for 24 hours during the day. This continues for 5 post-operative nights or as prescribed by the anaesthetist to reduce the risk of 3rd post-operative day MI.
- Doppler assessment of pedal pulses to check perfusion.
- Wean off intubation as able. Continue with nasal O2 as above.
- Observe for haemorrhage or haematoma at wound site.
- Monitor and record wound drainage.
- Monitor and record nasogastric drainage.
- Observe for mesenteric infarction or bowel obstruction. Report any abnormal abdominal distension, excessive nasogastric drainage or nausea or associated changes in haemodynamic status. Raised acidity of gastric juices may be indicative of bowel infarction.
- Care of patient with a urinary catheter — determine urine output is at least 30 ml/h.
- Maintain adequate hydration and blood pressure using i.v. crystalloids as prescribed until taking light diet.
- i.v. antibiotics as prescribed. Oral route when light diet is tolerated. Antibiotic cover given for 5 postoperative days.
- Repeat blood screening — FBC, U&Es, Hb.
- Reduce risk of DVT — passive leg exercises and SC heparin bd until fully mobile.
- Pre-op for patient anticoagulated using warfarin.
- Stop warfarin and commence heparin 2–3 days pre-op. Order fresh frozen plasma to have available if needed. For ladies on oestrogen pill, stop the pill 6 weeks prior to surgery.
- Analgesia via epidural catheter. Protect back and epidural site from trauma. Observe for leakage of CSF. Report immediately to medical team and anaesthetist any excessive patient discomfort, leakage of CSF, pyrexia, change in haemodynamic status, numbness or paralysis in lower limbs, or trauma at the site of epidural.
- Implement protocol for care of the patient with epidural continual infusion of analgesic and anti-emetic drugs.
- Assist with hygiene and mouth care until able to be self caring.

Return to ward when observations are stable
- Observations:
  Monitor and record vital signs 2–4 hourly.
  4 hourly obs for the next 48 hours or until stable for 24 hours.
  Reduce to tds, bd and daily by 7th day post op.

As able to tolerate — increase oral fluids, commencing with 30 ml/h then 60 ml, 90 ml, 120 ml and free fluids when bowel sounds are present. Regular mouth care until able to be self caring.

Cont'd

Check list cont'd

	Date	Signature
• Spigot NG tube when tolerating 60 ml per hour. If there is no nausea or vomiting and fluids continue to be tolerated, removed NG tube as instructed by medical team.		
• Move onto light diet meeting the requirement of any special diets when free fluids are tolerated.		
• Remove central line when no longer needed for CVP monitoring, route for hydration or antibiotics. Ensure tip of catheter is present on removal and send top to pathology for culture and sensitivity.		
• Mobilize bed to chair on 2nd or 3rd postoperative day as tolerated. Increase level of mobility each day, as tolerated. Aim for free mobility by 5th postoperative day.		
• Monkey pole over the patient's bed may aid independent movement whilst in bed.		
• Aid respiratory function by nursing in an upright position. Chest physio and deep breathing. Encourage patient to expectorate any phlegm and send any green phlegm for culture and sensitivity. If necessary and prescribed, administer antibiotics as prescribed.		
• Anticoagulant as prescribed. Encourage passive leg exercises to reduce the risk of DVT. Encourage patient not to cross legs.		
• Continued use of TEDS only if ABPI remains above 0.8 and no contraindication presents. Wash legs daily and check legs daily to ensure no ischaemic damage to tissues.		
• Remove wound drain after 24–48 hours or when exudate subsides as instructed by medical team.		
• Theatre dressing down on 3rd day.		
• Skin closures removed around 14th–17th postoperative day by community nurse if patient has been discharged.		
• Organize community care as assessed to be required by individual patients.		
• Health promotion.		
• Implement discharge plan — TTO's aspirin.		
• See in outpatients 4 weeks post discharge.		
• No driving until advised this is safe by consultant or GP, i.e. after postoperative assessment in outpatients clinic.		
• Advise not to carry anything heavier than a dinner tray for at least 4 weeks.		
• Advise to take a brisk walk as able each day and build up exercise tolerance gently, without overstretching abdominal muscles in the first 6 weeks.		
• Keep a balance between rest and gentle exercise.		
• Sexuality — allow the patient opportunity to discuss any concerns regarding sexuality. Alert medical staff to any patient concerns regarding erectile dysfunction so that referral can be made to a specialist clinic for advice and support as needed. Advise re ongoing healthy lifestyle issues to reduce the risk of further development of arterial disease.		

REFERENCES

MacSweeney S T R et al 1994 Smoking and the growth rates of small abdominal aortic aneurysms. Lancet 344: 651–652

Yusuf S W et al 1994 Transfemoral endoluminal repair of abdominal aortic aneurysm with bifurcated graft. Lancet 344: 650–651

FURTHER READING

Davis K 1990 Impotence after surgery (impotence following major pelvic surgery): nursing. Journal of Clinical Practice, Education and Management 4(18): 23–25

Caring for the patient undergoing carotid endarterectomy

CHAPTER 12

Cerebrovascular accident (CVA) accounted for 12% of deaths in 1991 in the UK (Health of the Nation 1992) and a high morbidity, that is, 100 000 strokes per year in the UK. This leaves patients dependent on others as a result of mental and/or physical handicaps. A 40% reduction in the incidence of CVA is the government's target for the year 2000. The incidence of occlusive CVA can be greatly reduced by changes in lifestyle, as outlined in Chapter 3. However, where there is established atheroembolic disease, surgical intervention in the form of carotid endarterectomy may be necessary to prevent CVAs. This should only be undertaken where the risk of peri-operative stroke remains less than 5%. The North American and European trials of comparing best medical and best surgical treatment demonstrated a 10–16-fold advantage for surgery in patients with a stenosis of greater than 70% (Smith 1996).

There is much debate about the pros and cons of screening for carotid occlusion and surgical intervention with its possible benefits or risks, as against the evidence of mortality and morbidity associated with medical treatment alone. Nevertheless, a study by Moore (1991) showed a steady reduction in the incidence of stroke between 1968 and 1981 that can be correlated with a similar increase in the number of carotid endarterectomies performed. According to this study, in 1968 no carotid endarterectomies were carried out in the area reviewed, but by 1981 the number of operations had increased to 32 per 100 000 population. The incidence of stroke death decreased over this period by 40%.

This chapter looks at the indications for surgical intervention, the procedure and the nursing management.

CAUSES OF CVA

Occlusion of the extracranial vasculature may lead to cell death in the structures served, notably the cerebral hemispheres and brain stem. However, owing to the anatomical structure of the Circle of Willis, blood flow may be sufficient to support brain tissue during the acute phase and thereby prevent chronic damage.

CVA commonly arises as a result of atheroma of the carotid system. Other causes include the following:

• Fibromuscular dysplasia, which is an uncommon condition affecting mostly women. It presents with areas of dilatation or stenosis, usually in the internal carotid, brought about by hyperplasia of the smooth muscle. The irregularity leads to thromboembolic disease and treatment is usually conservative, using antiplatelet agents such as aspirin. However, angioplasty may be indicated.

• Takayasu's arteritis, a form of giant cell arteritis usually affecting Asians, as described in Chapter 2. Treatment is usually with steroids but in severe cases cytotoxic agents may also be used.

• Dissecting aneurysm, which may be spontaneous or result from pressure associated with blunt trauma. It can result in sudden death. However, when patients survive, the carotid aneurysms that have formed can be supported by antiplatelet or anticoagulant medication, until in the majority of cases they resolve spontaneously. Occasionally reconstruction surgery may be required (Littooy 1979).

• Cervical radiation, used in the treatment of malignant conditions of the neck, can cause damage by scarring extracranial vessels and thus provoke atheroma formation.

Atherosclerosis of the extracranial carotid arteries is the major cause of CVA. Occlusion of the vessels may result from plaque stenosis or thromboembolism, the latter being more common.

Atherosclerotic plaques are frequently found at the bifurcation of vessels, where turbulence in blood flow aggravates the endothelial lining. This provokes the release of substances which stimulate platelet aggregation, and a proliferation of the smooth muscle cells in the medial layer of the vessel. Fatty streaks appear, and these eventually permeate the subendothelial layer of the vessel wall, where they develop into atheroma, creating a roughened luminal surface upon which thrombus collects; blood flow is significantly reduced. This may result in further narrowing of the vessel and eventually in total occlusion of blood flow.

If the atheroma becomes calcified it can be considered to be fairly stable. However, soft plaques, recognized as having a low density on ultrasound, are known to be associated with a high risk of cerebrovascular accident, owing to the instability of debris created by ulcer formation or haemorrhage within the plaque. This increases the risk of an embolic episode.

When an embolic episode is associated with platelet aggregation, this provokes the release of serotonin by the endothelial lining of the vessel lumen, so resulting in vasoconstriction and thus further reducing the lumen of the vessel and decreasing blood flow. The prostaglandin thromboxane A_2 is released as platelets come into contact with damaged endothelial tissue, and as this is a potent vasoconstrictor further reduction in the diameter of the vessel lumen results (Johnson & Anderson 1991). Disease of the carotid vessels may remain asymptomatic. However, in 15–20% of cases it may lead to transient ischaemic attacks (TIAs), which are by definition reversible, or cerebral infarction, which is not.

A symptom of *transient ischaemic attack* may be visual disturbance, typically a dulling of vision described by the patient as a blind being pulled down. This is known as amaurosis fugax. Other symptoms may include *monocular blindness, headache, hemiparesis, dizziness, ataxia or aphasia, all lasting for a maximum of 24 hours.* The duration of presenting symptoms in a single episode will determine the differential diagnosis between TIA and stroke.

The term *stroke* identifies a complex of symptoms and signs denoting brain damage. In the present context this brain damage is due to cerebral infarction associated with carotid thrombotic occlusion or an embolus arising from it, but may also be due to subarachnoid haemorrhage associated with hypertension or trauma, subdural haematoma—again caused by the trauma of head injury—embolus of cardiac origin or tumour.

CRITERIA FOR OPERATION

The criteria for proceeding to carotid endarterectomy are generally considered to be fulfilled when there is at least 70% stenosis of the diameter of the vessel in question, or when shaggy ulcerative plaques have been identified. Patients with asymptomatic but audible carotid disease on auscultation have a 3–5% chance of stroke, which is considerably higher than the risk of stroke as a complication of elective carotid endarterectomy (1–2%) (Hallet et al 1995). Surgery is not normally performed if the vessel is completely occluded, as the risk of subsequent subarachnoid haemorrhage from the sudden exposure of vessels to an unfamiliar, though normal, blood pressure is too great.

Persistent hypertension and continued smoking may also contraindicate elective surgery.

Opinion varies regarding the timing of endarterectomy after stroke in selected patients. Some authorities prefer a delay of at least 5 weeks after an acute incident because the stroke may still be evolving. Surgery following acute stroke can produce a normal or near-normal neurological examination in up to 40% of cases. It carries a 20% mortality rate, which is no worse than the prognosis for untreated stroke. The recurrent rate of stroke after carotid endarterectomy is 3–5%, with an 80% 5-year survival rate. Recurrence in untreated patients may vary from 25 to 60%.

REDUCING THE RISKS OF STROKE

Health promotion

It is important for the patient to be as fit as possible prior to admission; therefore support in stopping smoking, control of obesity, and reduction of excess alcohol intake and stress should be given.

Patients may require counselling to help them make an informed decision regarding the surgery proposed. They need to be aware of the risk of stroke, balancing this against the significant advantage of undergoing surgery rather than conservative management. The latter would address control of hypertension, raised serum lipids, diabetes, polycythaemia and thrombocytopaenia, smoking and platelet abnormalities.

It is not always easy for patients to comprehend clear information given to them in clinic if they are anxious or surprised by what has been said. Reinforcement of this information can be given by nursing staff and through clearly written literature that patients can take away and read at their own rate. A contact telephone number from which they can get further advice helps to support vascular patients.

Care should be taken to prevent sudden jerking of the patient's neck during transportation, investigations, intubation and surgery, to reduce the risk of an embolic episode.

PRE-OPERATIVE INVESTIGATIONS

The patient's general state of health needs to be defined, as well as specific investigations to determine the degree of stenosis and the morphology. Sources of emboli, e.g. cardiac, need to be elucidated.

Auscultation Turbulence around the bifurcation of the common carotid artery can be picked up clinically on auscultation and is detectable as a carotid bruit (noise). A bruit in the aortic arch or an aortic valve heart murmur may be transmitted to the carotid arteries; an ECG will help to determine its source.

An *ultrasound scan* (duplex) will safely determine the presence, position and degree of a stenosis and the morphology of a plaque.

Occasionally *angiography* and *digital subtraction angiography* may be required as part of the investigation, but as this carries a high risk of embolic incident it is used only as a last resort in some centres. Where cannulation can be performed via the aortic arch, the risk of dislodging thrombus in the carotid vessels is reduced.

Computed tomography (CT) or *magnetic resonance imaging (MRI)* can distinguish between cerebral infarction and other causes of neurological damage, as discussed

Pre-operative
investigations:

- duplex scan
- angiogram (possibly)
- chest X-ray
- electrocardiogram
- blood screening.

above, though stroke may not be evident for 12–24 hours after the event. Whilst MRI gives clear identification of infarction, CT is superior in identifying cerebral haemorrhage.

To ascertain general levels of fitness the following tests are performed:

- biochemical blood profile, a full blood count and serum lipids
- random blood sugar
- EEG; it is essential to determine that the signs which present are not due to intrinsic nervous disorders, e.g. epilepsy
- ECG
- chest X-ray
- pedal pulses, which may be checked as part of a general vascular assessment depending on suggestions of poor peripheral perfusion.

The results of these tests, which will be carried out in the outpatient department, will be given to patients should they wish to know them. The patient will return to the clinic to discuss the possibility of having a carotid endarterectomy if appropriate.

Patients undergoing carotid endarterectomy are usually admitted to hospital the day before surgery, when some of the tests may be repeated—for example, blood profile, full blood count. Grouping and cross-matching for two units of blood will be performed. On the day of surgery, the carotid duplex scan is repeated to establish an up-to-date clinical picture (Fig. 12.1)

Any pre-operative neurological deficits, including altered speech, paralysis of limbs, altered gait, facial weakness, difficulties with swallowing, visual disturbances and headaches, need to be recorded and communicated to the theatre and recovery nursing staff.

PREPARATION FOR THEATRE

The *anaesthetist* will visit the patient prior to surgery to assess suitability for anaesthesia. The usual information relating to allergies, previous deep vein thrombosis, reactions to anaesthetic gases and previous medical complaints will be gathered. A premedication may be prescribed, and any current antihypertensive medication should be given as usual pre-operatively, even though the patient may be nil by mouth.

Informed consent to the anaesthetic and the operation, including demonstration of an appropriate degree of understanding of the risks outlined in this chapter, will be obtained by the house officer.

If necessary, the neck will be shaved prior to theatre. Patients will be nil by mouth for 6 hours prior to surgery, *except for essential oral medication.*

Anti-embolic hosiery to reduce the risk of deep vein thrombosis is optional, depending on the state of arterial perfusion to the lower limbs and on consultant preference.

> Hypertensive medication should be administered pre-operatively as prescribed, even if patient is nil by mouth.

PERI-OPERATIVE PROCEDURE

Pressure relief

All vascular patients are liable to poor tissue perfusion and therefore carry an increased risk of pressure necrosis. Where possible, pressure relief devices should be used, and nursing intervention, by turning patients, should be implemented in theatre and at all stages of immobility.

Arterial lines

The insertion of an arterial line will allow continuous monitoring of blood pressure

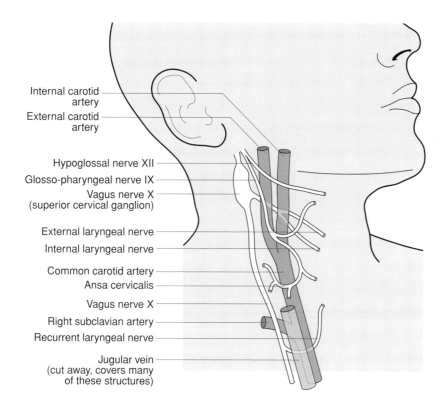

Fig. 12.1 The right carotid artery in relation to the surrounding nerves. The vagus (cranial nerve X) contains parasympathetic fibres; cervical sympathetic nerves also run through the superior cervical ganglion.

as well as providing access for arterial blood gas sampling and for the introduction of vasoactive drugs if haemodynamic stability is threatened.

Surgical technique

Following skin preparation, an incision is made into the sternomastoid muscle and a careful dissection is made to free the carotid at the bifurcation. It is essential not to dislodge loose debris within the lumen of the vessel and to avoid any damage to the surrounding nerves (Table 12.1).

Patients who would be unable to tolerate carotid clamping for long enough for the endarterectomy to be performed may benefit from the insertion of a temporary silicone shunt. Typically these patients are those with bilateral disease, with known disease in the Circle of Willis, with a past history of stroke and with peri-operative EEG abnormalities. Also, if the internal artery backflow pressure is less than 25–50 mmHg, shunting is required (Baker 1979). Long-term shunting may be indicated to prevent kinking and occlusion of vulnerable vessels. Risks associated with shunting are thromboembolus or air embolus. Visualization of the distal end of the vessel may be obstructed by the presence of a shunt.

The surgeon will next open the internal carotid artery and remove the atheroma (see Fig. 2.2).

The vessel is then closed, a vein or synthetic patch being used to prevent nar-

Table 12.1 Signs of damaged cranial nerves in the neck (after Brown 1987)

No.	Name	Consequence of injury
VII	Facial	Drooping lip and loss of smile
IX	Glossopharyngeal	Difficulty in swallowing
X	Vagus	
	—superior laryngeal	Difficulty swallowing, voice easily tired
	—recurrent laryngeal	Vocal cord paralysis, hoarseness
XI	Spinal accessory	Limited movement of neck and shoulder
XII	Hypoglossal	Affects the tongue—difficulty in speech and mastication
	Greater auricular branch of the brachial plexus	Paraesthesia of the face and ear

> A Taylor patch will reduce the risk of arteries narrowing during closing of vessel walls.

rowing of the vessel on closure. An antibacterial synthetic patch is currently being launched onto the market to reduce the risk of postoperative infection.

Determining adequate blood flow

Adequate blood flow may be simply determined by palpation of the vessel, but this technique does not always give sufficient accurate information regarding the status of blood flow and pressure.

Pressure of flow through the internal and external branches of the carotid can be ascertained prior to skin closure, with a sterile hand-held Doppler probe. The audible signal can help to determine the patency of the blood vessel. *Transcranial Doppler* may be performed to check for low flow or the presence of thrombus. Receptor pads are placed against the side of the head, enabling continuous monitoring of blood pressure. Some centres use *infra-red probes* to determine oxygen saturation. Where this is low, a shunt may be indicated.

An *on-table angiogram* is an efficient means of checking that no debris has been left or kinking occurred in the vessel prior to closure. If this is to be performed, an X-ray plate should be placed under the head and neck, prior to surgery, to avoid jerking and dislodgement of thrombus induced by setting up the investigation peri-operatively.

Incision closure

The wound in the side of the neck is usually about 12 cm long and is closed with a subcutaneous bead suture. A Redivac drain is inserted to reduce the risk of haematoma formation.

Depending on the site of incision, there may be a *permanently numb* area under the chin, which is caused by intra-operative trauma to small branches of the trigeminal nerve (fifth cranial nerve). The patient needs to be aware of this and to understand that care is needed when shaving.

POSTOPERATIVE CARE

The patient is transferred to a high-dependency unit until his or her condition has stabilized (usually after 24 hours).

Knowledge of the pre-operative baseline assessment of the vital signs will help in evaluating the stability of the patient's condition postoperatively. Continual monitoring and recording of vital signs and assessment of the tone of limbs, speech and swallowing will enable immediate action to be taken should complications arise, to reduce the long-term damage from an embolic event, haemorrhage, haematoma or infection.

Complications

Bradycardia

Changes in the pulse rate. As the baroreceptors will not have adjusted to the new blood pressures postoperatively, they will be over-responsive to the change, acting to reduce what is actually a normal pressure by slowing the heartbeat. The drop in pulse rate is a vagal response to the baroreceptors' sensitivity, and in order to prevent this phenomenon, a temporary vagal block is performed in theatre. It is therefore important to report to medical staff immediately if the pulse rate falls to less than 40 beats per minute. *Glycophyrrolate* 10–15 mcg per kilogram of body weight may be requested by the surgical or anaesthetic team to reduce the bradycardia.

> Postoperative observation
> —first 24 hours
> Observe for:
>
> - bradycardia (pulse rate < 40 beats/min)
> - tachycardia
> - abnormalities in BP
> - haemorrhage
> - loss of power in limbs
> - pupil reaction.

Hypertension

Hypertension may be the first sign of ruptured blood vessels, intracerebral haemorrhage or oedema as a cause of stroke. However, it may simply be a physiological response to pain, bladder distension, an uncomfortable position in bed or movement from one unit to another. It is therefore important not to give antihypertensive medication too quickly, and potentially increase the risk of hypotension. If, after addressing these issues, the blood pressure remains over 170/100 the medical team should be alerted. Antihypertensive medication and vasodilating drugs, such as nifedeipine, may then be prescribed.

Haematoma

Patients should be observed carefully for haemorrhage or haematoma at the wound site. As a precaution, *a stitch-cutter kept by the bed* will permit fast removal of the skin closure to release extreme pressure, caused by haematoma, on the vital structures in the neck.

If the airways become obstructed by haematoma—detectable by cyanosis, low oxygen saturation, stridor and laboured breathing or wheezing—an emergency tracheostomy will be performed. Drainage of wound exudate and haematoma will be aided by elevation of the head of the bed, postoperatively.

Hypotension

Haemorrhage may be indicated by a drop in blood pressure and a tachycardia. As the carotid is a major vessel, haemorrhage will quickly lead to collapse and should demand an immediate response. Colloids, blood transfusion vasoconstrictors, such as dopamine or dobutamine, may be needed to support the blood pressure. Return to theatre to control haemorrhage may be required.

Body temperature may increase by a few degrees as a normal response to the haemolysis of waste blood products during the postoperative period. However, should it rise above 37°C for more than 2 hours, medical staff should be informed and a cause of infection sought. The following should be checked for:

- wound infection
- chest infection
- deep vein thrombosis

- phlebitis at the site of the intravenous infusion
- other causes of infection, e.g. of the urinary tract.

Oxygen may be prescribed via a mask or nasal tubes after surgery, in order to assist the recovery of respiration following anaesthesia. This may be continued for up to 24 hours to reduce the risk of myocardial infarction. Oximetry will enable accurate continual assessment to be maintained.

Cerebrovascular accident

In spite of anticoagulants, peri-operative and postoperative embolus can create CVA.

Heparin may have been infused before the carotids were clamped during surgery. However, embolic debris from the site of the operation or new thrombus formation may become dislodged and lead to a stroke.

Other possible complications for which the patient needs routine observations are:

- decreased level of consciousness (The Glasgow Coma Scale may be used to assist in the assessment of neurological status if there appears to have been a cerebral insult and reduction in consciousness)
- loss of motor control
- changes in sensation to pain and/or touch
- dysphasia
- visual disturbances
- ipsilateral headache
- changes in the depth and rate of respiration.

Assessment of the swallowing reflex and weakness in the facial muscles also needs to be carried out at regular intervals.

Signs of damage to the cranial nerves in the neck are shown in Table 12.1.

Confusion

This may be caused by cerebral trauma, transient ischaemic attack, or electrolyte imbalance.

Deterioration in any of the vital signs needs to be reported to medical staff immediately. The interval of time between observations recorded is gradually spaced out but only if the above signs are stable.

Retention of urine

It is important to establish that the patient has passed urine postoperatively. Micturition may be inhibited in the early stages, because drugs used to control blood pressure may have included anticholinergics, which can cause urinary retention. Residual catheterization may be called for. If there is no hydration or elimination problem, there is no need to maintain a fluid balance chart.

It is usual to perform quarter-hourly observations for the first 12 hours, but the frequency of observations can be reduced, in line with a rising level of consciousness, over the next 24 hours.

Intravenous infusion

This is kept in place only until the patient is drinking and hydration is secure, unless i.v. antibiotics are being prescribed.

As soon as the patient feels able, he or she should be allowed to take oral fluids and then move on to light meals. However, this is contraindicated if the swallowing reflex has been lost owing to stroke, reduced level of consciousness or damage to the cranial nerves. Mastication may similarly be affected.

Care of the wound

A Redivac drain is sometimes inserted into the wound area to remove any postoperative haemorrhaging and to reduce the risk of haematoma formation. Drainage levels need to be recorded. It is not uncommon for the Redivac to be removed after the first 6–8 hours on the operative day if the drainage has reduced sufficiently, as it can serve as a port for potential infection.

The theatre dressing is taken down on the first postoperative day and only replaced if there are areas along the wound edge that have not united.

Control of pain and sickness

Minor discomfort is all that is usually experienced after this operation. One should aim to keep patients free from pain and any feeling of sickness. They need to be told to ask the nursing staff for analgesia and anti-emetics if necessary.

Postoperative passive leg exercises and deep breathing should be encouraged. Crossing the legs should be discouraged, as this increases the risk of deep vein thrombosis.

Mobilization

The patient may be mobilized from the first postoperative day, but subcutaneous anticoagulant drugs are normally administered as prescribed until full mobilization has been achieved.

Health promotion

If the risk recurrent stenosis is to be reduced, this is an integral part of care, as discussed in Chapter 3.

Discharge

Depending on the general well-being of the patient and the preference of the consultant, the patient may be discharged on the 3rd–5th postoperative day. Aspirin may be prescribed as a long-term prophylactic. Should a cerebral vascular accident have arisen, aspirin will only be prescribed providing the cause was thromboembolic, and not associated with cerebral haemorrhage. Antihypertensive medication may need to be adjusted postoperatively and the blood pressure monitored regularly by the Primary Health Care Team until stable and in the normal range.

Follow-up

It is common for patients to be asked to return to outpatients for a carotid scan 6 weeks after the operation. If there are continued indications of carotid disease in the contralateral vessel, ongoing duplex monitoring may be indicated until such time as further surgery becomes necessary.

SAMPLE CLINICAL GUIDELINES FOR THE CARE OF PATIENTS UNDERGOING CAROTID ENDARTERECTOMY

Check list

Action	Date	Signature

Critical pathway of care

- Following presentation of symptoms associated with carotid stenosis, e.g. blurred vision, headaches, dizziness, TIAs, CVA
- Carotid scan is requested if this has not been already done by the general practitioner
- Referral to vascular surgeon if carotid stenosis present
- Seen in clinic by consultant
- Blood screening:
  Full blood count
  Lipids/cholesterol
  Urea and electrolytes
- If scan needed to be requested during first OPD appointment, return to OPD two weeks later for results
- Decision to operate is made by consultant with patient
- Patient information re carotid endarterectomy and healthy lifestyle

Added to waiting list

Admitted to the ward

- Routine nursing and medical assessments including discharge assessment of needs.
- Note any muscle weakness, headaches, loss of taste or difficulties with swallowing; speech and vision are noted.
- Alert all staff, including porters and technicians to the need to support the patient's neck when transferring and to prevent jarring which may dislodge debris.
- BP and pulse as baseline observations.
- Repeat carotid scan on day of surgery.
- Chest X-ray.
- ECG.
- Blood screen.
- Cross-match only
  or group and save 2 units of blood depending on local policy.
- Consent to anaesthetic and surgery.
- Shave neck if required.
- Prep for theatre.
- Pre-med if prescribed.
- Anti-embolic stockings if requested by consultant, to reduce risk of DVT where there is no evidence of arterial insufficiency to the lower limbs on Doppler assessment (ABPI greater than 0.8).
- Give oral medication even if nil by mouth pre-operatively, especially anti-hypertensive drugs.

First 24 hours postoperatively

- Transferred to a high-dependency unit until condition has stabilized (usually after 24 hours).

Cont'd

Check list cont'd

Action	Date	Signature

- Continual monitoring for the first 24 hours postoperative. To include recording of:
  - — ECG, BP, pulse (immediately report to medical staff — pulse less than 40, BP < 100/50 > 170/100)
  - — (Glycophyrrolate 10–15 mcg/kg body weight may be requested by the surgical or anaesthetic team to reduce the bradycardia.)
- Temperature, respiration.
- O2 saturation.
- Continual nasal O2 as prescribed for 24 hours (possibly humidified).
- Hourly observation to assess function of limbs, swallowing reflex, weakness in facial muscles for first 12 hours.
- If there is any signs of a cerebral insult proceed with neurological assessment using the Glasgow scale.
- If all remains stable, reduce frequency of observations with rising level of consciousness over the forthcoming 24 hours.
- Observe for haemorrhage or haematoma at wound site.
- Drains may be removed from site 6–8 hours postoperatively at the surgeon's request as drainage reduces or stops. Early and appropriate removal will help to reduce the risk of infection through the drainage ports.
- Monitor wound dressing for strike through of exudate.
- Determine patient has passed urine postoperatively.
- Commence i.v. antibiotics as prescribed.
- Repeat blood screening — FBC, U&Es.
- Check for numbness in face, tongue and difficulty in swallowing prior to giving fluids and solids orally.
- Normal diet and oral fluids as soon as tolerated.

When returned to the ward postoperatively

- Return to ward when observations or vital signs are stable.
- Reduce observations of vital signs and motor control to 2–4 hourly when stable for 24 hours.
- 4 hourly obs from 24–48 hours or until stable for 24 hours.
- Reduce to tds, bd and daily by 3rd day post op.
- Remove IVI when hydration is stable — usually around 24 hours post op.
- Mobilize first postoperative day if stable.
- Commence subcutaneous anticoagualants as prescribed.
- Theatre dressing down after 24 hours. Leave wound open if dry.
- Skin closures removed on 5th postoperative day.
- Health promotion to reduce the risk of recurrent arterial disease.
- Implement discharge plan
- TTOs to include aspirin providing there are no contraindications.
- Repeat carotid scan 6 weeks postoperatively, then see in clinic with results.

REFERENCES

Baker W H 1979 Diagnosis and treatment of carotid artery disease. Futura, Mount Kisco, N.Y.

Brown S 1987 Practical points in the assessment and care of the patient having a carotid endarterectomy. Journal of Post Anaesthetic Nurse 2: 41–42

Hallet J W Jnr et al 1995 Handbook of patient care in vascular surgery. Little, Brown, Boston

Health of the Nation 1992 A summary of the strategy for health in England. HMSO, London

Johnson S, Anderson B 1991 Carotid endarterectomy: a review. Critical Care Nursing Clinics of North America 3(3): 499–506

Littooy R 1979 Cerebral vascular insufficiency: understanding and recognition. In: Baker W H (ed) Diagnosis and treatment of carotid artery disease. Futura, Mount Kisco, N.Y.

Moore W S 1991 Vascular surgery: a comprehensive review. Saunders, Philadelphia

Smith S 1996 Safety in carotid surgery. Unpublished paper presented to the Society of Vascular Nurses, September 1996, Birmingham

FURTHER READING

Moore W S 1993 Carotid endarterectomy for prevention of stroke. Western Journal of Medicine 159(1): 37–43

Strandness D E 1993 Carotid endarterectomy: current status and effect of clinical trials. Cardiovascular Surgery 1(4): 311–316

Thompson J E et al 1993 Carotid endarterectomy. Advances in Surgery 26: 99–131

Therapies

Treatments in common use in vascular surgery

All qualified nurses are called upon to dispense drugs and are therefore expected to possess a working knowledge of their actions and side-effects. Prescribing by nurses is increasing. This chapter highlights some of the groups of drugs associated with the treatment of peripheral vascular disorders and is intended for use as a ready reference. For further details the practitioner is advised to consult the *British National Formulary*.

CARDIOVASCULAR DRUGS

Drugs used in hypertension

Diuretics

Fluid removal with diuretics is effected through the kidneys (Table 13.1). Diuretics are especially useful for removing the fluid retention caused by heart failure, particularly pulmonary oedema. They are relatively ineffective for other forms of oedema such as postural ankle swelling, and so are not a convenient alternative to elevation or compression. *Thiazides* (e.g. bendrofluazide) are mild but generally long-acting. *Metolazone* is a uniquely powerful new thiazide and must be carefully monitored in respect to hypotension and dehydration. *Loop* diuretics such as *frusemide* are more potent and have a speedy onset of action. Both groups allow removal of potassium from the body.

Potassium-sparing diuretics such as amiloride and spironolactone are mild when used alone but especially useful in combination with any of the above (e.g. co-amilofruse). Elderly patients are sensitive to loss of potassium, particularly if they

Table 13.1 Diuretics

Type	Features	Problems
Thiazides	Mild; useful where rapid diuresis not tolerated	K$^+$ loss Hypotensive effect Impaired GTT
Loop, e.g. frusemide, bumetanide	Rapid, effective; can be given in high doses for renal failure	K$^+$ loss Hypotension, nausea, gout, impaired GTT (frusemide)
Potassium-sparing	Mild; useful in hypokalaemia	Can be ineffective alone GI disturbances, hyperkalaemia, gynaecomastia (spironolactone)
Combination	Effective; relatively safe for long-term use	As for individual compounds

also take digoxin, so potassium monitoring is helpful. Such combination diuretics tend to have superseded potassium supplements nowadays.

Beta-blockers

Beta-adrenergic blockers block the effects of the sympathomimetics at the beta receptors, which are present in the heart, peripheral vessels and bronchi (Table 13.2).

The effect of beta-blockers is to slow the heart rate, protecting it against sudden surges in adrenergic activity provoked by stress. The excitability of the heart is depressed, so cardiac output is reduced and the heart does less work (a so-called negative inotropic effect). Beta-blockers are therefore effective for hypertension, because they reduce cardiac output and lower pulse rate, and for angina, because they reduce the heart's capacity for work.

Side-effects vary somewhat between different drugs. *Bronchospasm* occurs because beta$_2$ activity, which causes bronchodilatation, is blocked. Some drugs are effective against beta$_1$ receptors only and are said to be cardioselective, but this selectivity is only relative. One should beware of using them for asthmatics.

Tiredness and *somnolence* occur mainly with those beta-blockers that are lipid-soluble and cross the blood–brain barrier. Because the capacity for cardiac work is reduced, *heart failure* may occur, and care should therefore be taken with patients who have a history of this.

Most importantly, in the context of this book, beta-blockers can cause profound *vasoconstriction*, which may be severe enough to cause *critical ischaemia* in the patient with peripheral vascular disease. Effects are dose-related.

Table 13.2 Beta-blockers

Drug	Features	Problems
Propranolol Metoprolol Atenolol Labetolol	Reduces BP Reduces cardiac output Protects against angina and MI	Bronchospasm, cardiac failure, peripheral ischaemia

Angiotensin-converting enzyme (ACE) inhibitors

ACE converts angiotensin I to angiotensin II. Inhibition therefore reduces blood pressure (Table 13.3).

Table 13.3 ACE inhibitors

Drug	Features	Problems
Enalapril Captopril Lisinopril	Reduces BP Helps heart failure Useful for diabetics	Hypotension (with thiazides), hyperkalaemia, renal failure, headache, cough

ACE inhibitors are particularly useful for diabetics because they have a protective effect against diabetic nephropathy.

Adding an ACE inhibitor to a thiazide can produce a profound reduction in blood pressure. It is therefore essential to stop the diuretic, start the ACE inhibitor and then slowly reintroduce the diuretic.

Heart failure may be treated with ACE inhibitors. This treatment may be in conjunction with digoxin and diuretics. Low doses are usually effective.

Side-effects include hypotension, hyperkalaemia (it is dangerous to combine them with potassium-sparing diuretics), renal failure, headaches and, not uncommonly, an irritating dry cough.

Calcium antagonists

These drugs have the effect of reducing the activity of cardiac muscle cells and some smooth muscle cells by blocking the system for transporting calcium into them (Table 13.4). This lowers excitability in the heart (thus slowing conduction), reduces the contractility of cardiac muscle fibres (so reducing cardiac output) and reduces the tone of arteriolar smooth muscle.

In functional terms, therefore, cardiac arrhythmias such as paroxysmal tachycardias are reduced through the delaying action on the conduction system. Conversely, arrhythmias associated with degrees of heart block are made worse.

Blood pressure is reduced because of lower cardiac output and decreased peripheral resistance. Angina is treated by reducing cardiac work and vasodilating the coronary vessels. Calcium antagonists are the drug of choice in crescendo angina, as they reduce the risk of myocardial infarction.

The clinician has to be aware of the balance of effects. Reduced cardiac output can result in heart failure. Heart block can be precipitated.

Different calcium antagonists have variations in their degree of effect. Thus *verapamil* is useful for the arrhythmias and *nifedipine* for angina. New drugs are being developed that produce less peripheral vasodilatation, which can cause unacceptable flushing.

Other side-effects include headaches, dizziness and ankle oedema (unrelated to heart failure).

For the peripheral vascular patient, calcium antagonists are a relatively safe treatment for angina or hypertension. *Nifedipine* and related drugs are also effective in Raynaud's phenomenon.

Table 13.4 Calcium antagonists

Drug	Features	Problems
Verapamil	Used for angina, hypertension, arrhythmias	Heart failure, heart block, flushing, headache, dizziness
Nifedipine	Used for angina, hypertension, Raynaud's	Flushing, headache, dizziness
Amlodipine Diltiazem	Used for angina, arrhythmias, hypertension	As above

Nitrates and vasodilators

Nitrates

Nitrates are powerful vasodilators, especially of the coronary system (Table 13.5). They also reduce venous return, cardiac work and output. All these effects are useful in angina but they are not of benefit in peripheral vascular disease.

Glyceryl trinitrate (GTN) is in common use sublingually as the immediate treatment for acute angina. Its effect is speedy (within 5 minutes) and lasts for 20–30 minutes. It is also available as a spray, which has the advantage of a long shelf life (even in one's pocket), against the 8 weeks' life of tablets in a bottle. There is also an intravenous preparation for hospital use.

Long-acting variations on GTN are commonly used for the prophylaxis of angina, e.g. GTN transdermal patches, sustained-release GTN, isosorbide mononitrate and dinitrate. Tolerance to topical GTN may develop.

Table 13.5 Nitrates

Drug	Features	Problems
GTN	Treatment of acute angina	Headache, flushing, dizziness, hypotension, tachycardia
Long-acting GTN	Prophylaxis of angina	As above, but generally better tolerated

Other vasodilators

While there is good evidence that nifedipine (above) produces significant vasodilatation, there is little evidence, according to the *British National Formulary* (1996), that other drugs in this category have any beneficial effect in peripheral vascular disease, with the exception of prazosin and thymoxamine.

Nevertheless, products in this class have been highly promoted by their manufacturers and patients with peripheral vascular disease may well enter hospital taking one or more of them (Table 13.6).

Table 13.6 Other vasodilators

Drug	Features	Problems
Prazosin	Alpha-adrenergic blocking agent Indicated for Raynaud's	Postural hypotension, palpitation
Thymoxamine	For Raynaud's	Diarrhoea, flushing, headaches
Naftidrofuryl Nicotinic acid, etc. Cinnarizine Oxpentifylline	Said to have vasodilator properties	Efficacy unproven

Sympathomimetics

These drugs are so called because they have a positive effect on the peripheral receptors of the sympathetic nervous system (Table 13.7). There are three types of receptor:

- beta$_1$ receptors
- beta$_2$ receptors
- alpha receptors.

A beta$_1$ receptor's action affects the heart muscle, increasing the rate and/or contractility of the heart. This is known as a positive inotropic effect. Though this is often a desired effect, it may be dangerous in people with angina or heart failure because of the extra work the heart has to do.

Beta$_2$ receptor sympathomimetics act on the peripheral circulation to produce vasodilatation. Their effect is usually on those vessels supplying muscles and the vital organs rather than the skin.

Alpha receptor sympathomimetics cause vasoconstriction. The effect that this has on the skin is of particular concern for the vascular patient.

Sympathomimetic drugs rarely have pure beta$_1$, beta$_2$ or alpha effects. The overlap determines which drugs are used for which purpose.

Beta-adrenergic drugs (beta-agonists)

These include isoprenaline, dobutamine, dopamine and dopexamine. Isoprenaline is used as a temporary treatment for heart block and Stokes-Adams attacks, though these conditions are treated long-term nowadays with a pacemaker.

Dobutamine particularly improves renal blood flow at low doses, and so affords good protection in low output states such as cardiogenic shock, or heart failure associated with myocardial infarction or cardiomyopathy. Dopamine may also be used in this way. In higher doses dobutamine is used deliberately to stress the heart during a thallium scan (as opposed to using a treadmill).

Alpha-agonists

These have only limited use. The vasoconstriction is used to elevate the blood pressure, but the adverse effect on perfusion through tissues, such as the kidneys, makes their use hazardous. Nevertheless, alpha-agonists are used in hypotension that may complicate spinal or epidural anaesthesia (spinal shock), because the hypotension is due to sympathetic block. Drugs in this category include ephedrine, metaraminol and noradrenaline. Side-effects include a dry mouth and restlessness.

Table 13.7 Sympathomimetics

Drug	Features	Problems
Beta-agonists Isoprenaline Dobutamine	Positive inotropic effect Vasodilator (at low doses)	Can cause angina or heart failure
Alpha-agonists Ephedrine Metaraminol	Used to correct acute hypotension	May cause ischaemia of vital organs

Drugs associated with clotting

Fibrinolytics and anticoagulants

For a full account of fibrinolytics and anticoagulants (Tables 13.8, 13.9), see Chapter 9 on critical ischaemia.

Table 13.8 Fibrinolytic drugs

Drug	Features	Problems
Streptokinase Urokinase	Immediate production of plasmin i.v. or intra-arterial injection	Bleeding Allergy Anaphylaxis
rt-PA	As above	Bleeding

Table 13.9 Anticoagulants

Drug	Features	Problems
Heparin	Rapid onset Standard—i.v. only	Bleeding Hypersensitivity—not for long-term use
	Low molecular weight— SC (prophylactic)	(thrombocytopaenia)
Warfarin Phenindione	Long-term use Oral	Bleeding Hypersensitivity and drug interactions (warfarin) Needs regular INR

Antiplatelet drugs

It is now common practice to use *aspirin* as prophylaxis against thromboembolic disease in the coronary, cerebral and peripheral circulations (Table 13.10). If started immediately after myocardial infarction it reduces mortality during the first month. Its routine use after bypass surgery has been advocated.

The mode of action is the reduction of platelet aggregation; it thus undermines part of the mechanism of thrombus formation. Doses as low as 75 mg daily are thought to be sufficient for this purpose.

It must, however, be remembered that gastrointestinal side-effects are recorded even at this low dosage, and that aspirin can provoke asthma. Soluble and enteric-coated forms are reputed to reduce the gastrointestinal effects.

Dipyridamole is an alternative to aspirin, developed for use as an adjunct to anticoagulants in protecting patients with prosthetic valves.

Epoprostenol inhibits platelet aggregation and is also a potent vasodilator. It has a very short half-life, so it is mainly given by i.v. infusion during renal dialysis.

LIPID-LOWERING DRUGS

Hypercholesterolaemia is a prominent risk factor in the aetiology of coronary vascular disease and peripheral vascular disease. The treatment is dietary restriction.

Table 13.10 Antiplatelet drugs

Drug	Features	Problems
Aspirin	Cheap and effective	Peptic ulcers and gastric irritation Asthma
Dipyridamole	Useful second line where aspirin not tolerated	Hypotension (rare after recent MI or angina) Headache
Epoprostenol	i.v. keeps renal patients' shunts open	Half-life 3 min

Only where this fails or is insufficient are lipid-lowering drugs utilized (Table 13.11).

Bile acids facilitate the absorption of cholesterol from the gut, and binding these acids reduces absorption. *Cholestyramine* is a bile-acid binding agent. It is given in the form of a powder, which is taken with meals.

Clofibrate and associated drugs directly reduce cholesterol in the blood, but side-effects are quite common and include nausea, vomiting and anorexia. Gallstones may be produced.

The statins (simvastatin, etc.) competitively inhibit a coenzyme vital to the production of cholesterol in the body. They also can cause nausea, as well as headaches and flatulence.

Fish oils are used to lower triglycerides but are less effective against cholesterol.

Table 13.11 Lipid-lowering agents

Drug	Features	Problems
Cholestyramine	Lowers dietary absorption of cholesterol	Inconvenient
Bezafibrate Clofibrate Simvastatin Fish oil preparations Nicotinic acid	Interferes with metabolism of cholesterol and triglycerides	Commonly nausea and other gastrointestinal symptoms Gallstones (clofibrate)

STEROIDS

Corticosteroids

Steroids and operations

During acute stress the body's production of cortisol increases from 20 mg/24 h to up to 300 mg/24 h. The return to normal levels is generally fairly rapid.

For people who take long-term steroids and whose adrenal glands are suppressed and cannot mount a quick response to stress, the best course is to administer 100 mg hydrocortisone, i.v. or i.m., pre-operatively (Table 13.12). This is repeated every 8 hours for 24 hours, and the daily dose is then halved on alternate days, down to 20–30 mg/day. If the patient is receiving oral medication by this time, the dose of prednisolone is similarly reduced to the usual dose. The conversion factor is: *1 mg prednisolone is equivalent to 4 mg hydrocortisone.*

As adrenal suppression may persist for several years after steroids have been stopped, and this may only be evident during stress, anaesthetists must be informed about steroid medication even if it was stopped years before.

Side-effects of steroids

It is always necessary to balance the benefits of steroid use against the problems incurred. Short-term use—e.g. a 1-week treatment for an acute attack of asthma—is virtually without side-effects.

The vascular patient may be taking steroids for a variety of reasons, such as:

- unassociated disease, e.g. asthma, Addison's disease
- disease which may have vascular complications, e.g. rheumatoid arthritis, polyarteritis nodosa.

Also, prednisolone therapy may provoke side-effects with vascular consequences, such as diabetes and osteoporotic fractures.

Some of the important side-effects of steroid therapy are as follows:

- Osteoporosis. This produces bone pain which, particularly in the elderly, can lead to immobilizing back and leg pain. It is a differential diagnosis of claudication and can coexist with it. The condition is more severe if fractures occur, characteristically in the back or hip. A separate side-effect, unrelated to osteoporosis, is avascular necrosis of the head of the femur, in which the bone is simply starved; the only treatment is hip replacement.
- Muscle wasting. This can complicate the above.
- Diabetes, as steroids raise blood sugars.
- Increased susceptibility to infection. This is due to adrenal suppression, which prevents an increase in steroid levels in response to stress. Any infection in the patient who takes long-term steroids requires a temporary increase in the dose.
- Hypertension. This is due to the sodium and fluid-retaining attributes of mineralocorticoids. Blood pressure readings need to be monitored frequently, particularly if the patient is already hypertensive when steroids are started, or if the dose of steroids is being altered.
- Peptic ulceration.

Table 13.12 Steroids

Drug	Features	Problems
Prednisolone, hydrocortisone and all steroids with a predominantly glucocorticoid effect	Suppress inflammatory response to asthma, rheumatoid arthritis, infections, etc.	Multiple side-effects as above Must not be withdrawn suddenly

- Withdrawal symptoms, which may be minor (rhinorrhoea, conjunctivitis, arthralgia), severe (adrenal suppression, hypotension) or major, resulting in death. Patients on steroids should carry a card which displays the up-to-date dose.

Anabolic steroids

Anabolic steroids are used in the treatment of lipodermatosclerosis and in the management of vascular manifestations of Behçet's disease (Table 13.13).

Anabolic steroids have protein-building properties, but should only be used with great caution and are not recommended for women who are premenopausal. Side-effects may include masculinization, headache, dyspepsia, hair loss, euphoria, depression and cramp. Cholestatic jaundice has also been reported.

Table 13.13 Anabolic steroids

Drug	Features	Problems
Stanozolol	Reduces lipodermatosclerosis	Masculinization, headache, dyspepsia, hair loss, euphoria, depression, cramp, cholestatic jaundice

DEXTRANS

These are macromolecular substances which stay in this form long enough for them to expand the plasma volume (Table 13.14). They will not pass through cell membranes and exert a strong osmotic pressure, drawing fluid into the plasma. This is particularly useful when plasma loss has been sudden and has included loss of plasma protein (e.g. haemorrhage or burns). Dextrans are therefore to be considered as a suitable holding measure when blood is required but not yet available. Dextran 70 is used for this purpose.

Dextran 40 has a lower molecular weight and is used for a different purpose: to help preserve the circulation in critically ischaemic legs before surgery and as prophylaxis against thromboembolic disease after surgery.

Side-effects include bleeding, hypersensitivity reactions, and fluid overload which can possibly lead to heart failure, especially in the elderly. Central venous pressure and interference with blood grouping should be monitored. Infusion should therefore be set up after blood is taken if possible.

Table 13.14 Dextrans

Drug	Features	Problems
Dextran 70	Replaces blood volume in haemorrhage and burns	Bleeding Cardiac failure Problems with cross-matching
Dextran 40	Permeates thrombosed blood vessels	

ANALGESICS

The two main simple analgesics (Table 13.15) for mild to moderate pain, particularly of a neuromuscular nature, are aspirin and paracetamol.

Table 13.15 Analgesics

Drug	Features	Problems
Non-opiate analgesics	Mild; available over the counter (OTC)	Aspirin: GI bleeds Paracetamol: dangerous in overdose
Combination analgesics	Stronger than paracetamol alone; some available OTC	As above
Opiates	Powerful in oral or parenteral form	Hypotension, respiratory depression, addiction

Aspirin

This has anti-inflammatory properties and is chemically related to some of the non-steroidal anti-inflammatory drugs. It is also an antipyretic.

Drawbacks include a tendency to gastric irritation. Preparations designed to prevent this effect include soluble and enteric-coated versions. Aspirin also interacts with a number of other drugs; for example, it *potentiates* the effect of other analgesics, NSAIDs, anticoagulants, phenytoin and valproate. Metoclopramide and other anti-emetics potentiate its action. Allergy to aspirin is not uncommon. The effect of aspirin as an antiplatelet drug is catalogued above.

Paracetamol

This is as efficacious as aspirin but is a weaker antipyretic, with no anti-inflammatory action. It has fewer side-effects and does not irritate the stomach. The one problem associated with its easy availability is that an overdose causes delayed damage to the liver which can be fatal. Treatment is with intravenous acetylcysteine and must be commenced within 12 hours. There are literally hundreds of over-the-counter preparations containing asprin and/or paracetamol. In common medical use there are mixtures with opiates such as co-dydramol (dihydrocodeine and paracetamol) and co-proxamol (dextropropoxyphene and paracetamol).

Stronger analgesics

Those in common use are mainly opioids. As they are stronger, they may be combined with paracetamol, for example, to provide the moderately potent combinations referred to above. They can, however, cause drowsiness, nausea, vomiting and constipation and, in higher doses, respiratory depression or hypotension. Many are controlled drugs because of their addictive effects.

Opioids compete with one another for the same receptors on nerve cells. Thus an opioid with a weak analgesic action may partially inhibit the effect of a strong one. For this reason buprenorphine may actually cause withdrawal symptoms in heroin addicts.

Morphine and diamorphine are the usual drugs of choice for severe pain. 10 mg of morphine is equivalent to 5 mg of diamorphine. Delayed release morphine is available, administered twice in 24 hours. A morphine elixir may be prescribed for breakthrough pain.

Codeine and dihydrocodeine are weaker than the above but cause fewer dependency problems and are more suitable for day-to-day use. *Dextropropoxyphene* is only effective with paracetamol. *Buprenorphine* has a long half-life and is used as a twice daily dose, sublingually, for chronic pain.

Fentanyl has a short half-life and is useful for epidural anaesthesia with local anaesthetics for epidural blocks.

Pethidine is milder and shorter-acting than morphine, and so is used intra- and postoperatively.

Tramadol is a new oral opiate. Evidence from abroad suggests that it might be of use, though the experience with it here is still being evaluated.

WOUND CARE

Patients who present with peripheral vascular disease have a high risk of developing complications in wound healing, as the underlying pathology is not conducive to this. It is a prudent nurse who realizes this and produces a holistic assessment and plan of care for the patient.

Wounds should be cleansed by gentle irrigation with a warmed cleansing solution. While it is important not to disturb newly formed epithelial cells, it is equally important to ensure that all debris, including exudate, slough, foreign bodies and previously used wound care products, are removed thoroughly before the application of new dressings.

Postoperative interventions should be aimed at preserving blood flow to maintain tissue oxygen perfusion and nutritional requirements for effective collagen synthesis, angiogenesis and the prevention of infection (Ting 1991). Although it is recognized that epidermal repair is enhanced by an oxygen-rich environment, it is also known that the creation of a hypoxic environment—for example, by the use of hydrocolloid dressing—speeds up angiogenesis (Cherry et al 1985). Miller (1994) suggests that it may therefore be more appropriate to use a hydrocolloid dressing to deslough a wound and to promote angiogenesis in the destructive and proliferative phase. However, the use of a semipermeable dressing that allows oxygen to penetrate may be more appropriate when promoting epithelialization.

Wounds need protecting from adverse internal and external environments. For the patient who is incontinent or who perspires heavily, carefully chosen dressings will provide protection. Trauma that may be caused by the entry of infection or foreign bodies such as particles of cotton wool, gauze and wound dressings needs to be avoided if wound healing is not to be delayed (Johnson 1988). It is equally important to protect the skin surrounding a wound, and the use of an absorbent dressing and emollients may prevent excoriation from exudate.

The ideal temperature for wound healing has been demonstrated to be around 35°C. Therefore, where possible, dressings should only be removed when it is really necessary, as during dressing changes the temperature has been seen to drop to around 25°C. This will reduce leucocyte activity and the ability of blood to convey oxygen to the tissues. It can take up to 40 minutes for the wound's temperature to recover after a change of dressing, and 3 hours for mitosis to return to normal (Myres 1982).

It has been shown that wounds heal up to 40% more quickly in a moist environment. This may be due to the fact that the migration of endothelial cells is not inhibited by dry fibrous eschar. In a moist environment macrophages have been found to be more prolific than neutrophils. This is important, as macrophages are more phagocytic than neutrophils, stimulate angiogenesis and are responsible for the formation of fibroblasts. Collagen, which is the structural protein laid down by fibroblasts, forms the matrix for wound repair; dressings which allow for this include hydrocolloids, hydrogels, alginates, foams and vapour-permeable films.

A further advantage of maintaining a moist environment is that dressing changes will be less painful, and less trauma will be caused to the epithelializing wound bed if the dressing does not adhere to the wound.

There is some evidence that wounds heal better in a slightly acidic environment of around pH 6. A hydrocolloid environment meets this requirement, whereas dressings which are permeable produce a pH of above 7.

Knowledge of dressings formerly used will help to determine the choice of dressings. Any previously known allergies to dressings should be considered and the product avoided (Fig. 2.4; Table 13.16).

Table 13.16 Common allergens

Allergen	Type	Source of allergen
Balsam of Peru/Fragrance Mix	Perfumes	Some medicaments
Cetylstearyl alcohol	Vehicle	Aqueous cream, corticosteroid creams, emulsifying ointment, Flamazine, Hioxyl, Ichthopaste bandages, Viscopaste bandages
Ester gum resin	Adhesive	Some bandages and sticking plaster
Gentamycin	Antibiotic	Cream and ointment
Framycetin	Antibiotic	Framycetin gauze dressing (Sofra-Tulle)
Neomycin	Antibiotic	Neomycin cream and Cicatrin
Parabenz	Preservative	Paste bandages, e.g. Icthaband, Viscopaste, Zincaband and some medicaments
Penosept	Preservative	Calaband paste bandages
Rubber mixes	Rubbers	Stockings, Tubigrip, some bandages, e.g. cohesive bandages
Wool alcohols	Lanolin	Found in many emollients, e.g. E45 and Oilatum

Dressings should not be left in place for longer than the recommended time for each product. However, it is better to leave the wound undisturbed for several days if possible. Should exudate strike through, it is better to change the dressing to avoid the penetration of microbes. Heavily exuding wounds may need a daily dressing at the early stage of healing.

When selecting a product for individual wounds it is important to bear in mind that a product is only effective if used for the purpose for which it was intended. It is therefore advisable to follow the manufacturer's instructions closely. Table 13.17 lists some commonly used wound care products.

Wounds should be assessed at each dressing change, and the effectiveness of the product and the status of the wound should be evaluated. Wounds are not static, and the nurse needs to respond according to the stage of wound healing and the presentation of the wound bed.

The characteristics of an ideal dressing that will enhance wound healing are outlined in Box 7.1.

Table 13.17 Examples of wound care products

Status of wound	Suggested products
Clean incisional line	Mefix surgical dressing
	Occlusive dressings
	Low adherent gauze
	Non-adherent silicone viscose dressing
Exudating wound	Alginate
	Occlusive
	Foam
	Hydrocellular dressing
	Hydrocolloid
Clean granulating wound, low exudate or dry	Hydrogel
	Non-adherent, silicone viscose dressing
	Foam
	Hydrocellular
Epithelializing	Non-adherent, viscose silicone dressing
	Hydrogel
Necrotic	Enzymatic agent
	Hydrogel
	Occlusive
Sloughy	Enzymatic agent
	Hydrogel
	Hydrocolloid
	Hioxyl cream
	Occlusive
	Semi-occlusive dressings
Infected	Systemic antibiotics to wound bed in conjunction with local wound-care products, e.g.
	Flamazine (*Pseudomonas*)
	Iodine-based dressings
MRSA	Check for infection and treat accordingly; Bactroban may be indicated, depending on size of wound and frequency of dressing change
	Iodoflex/Iodosorb/Inodine
Fungating	Metrotop
Malodorous	Actisorb, silver-impregnated carbon dressing
	Lyofoam C
	Katlicarb
	Non-occlusive dressings
	Hydrogel
Overgranulating	Overgranulation may resolve without treatment; otherwise consider:
	Silver nitrate
	Light steroids on prescription only
	Non-occlusive dressings
Bath emollients	Hydromol
	Oilatum
Emollients to protect surrounding skin, especially for leg ulcer patients	50% liquid paraffin with 50% white paraffin
	Vaseline
	Aqueous cream
	Hydromol cream
	Zinc and castor oil
	E45
	Unguentum Merck
	Paraffin tulle dressings
Leg ulcers	Primary dressings as above, depending on need
	Paste bandages
	Viscopaste
	Icthopaste
	Setopaste
	Bandage: choice depends on aetiology (see Table 13.18)
	NB: *Compression should only be used where there are no indications of ischaemia or other contraindications*

Bandage classifications

Bandage classifications are presented in Table 13.18.

Class 1

These are used mainly for retention of dressings. Sub-bandage pressure does not exceed a few mmHg. Class 1 bandages are usually composed of lightweight elastomeric threads that give a high degree of elasticity.

Class 2

This group of bandages gives support without compression. They are not very extensible, as they have limited elastomeric fibres, and they are therefore suitable for supporting joints and preventing the formation of oedema. They will not reduce oedema that already exists. Sub-bandage compression is only a few mmHg, as for class 1. However, if they are used in conjunction with a paste bandage, up to 20 mmHg sub-bandage pressure can be achieved during exercise owing to the cohesion of the paste bandage and the elastocrepe.

Class 3

Class 3 comprises compression bandages, which are divided into four groups, as listed below. Compression bandages are graded according to their ability to maintain predetermined levels of tension under controlled laboratory conditions. This tension determines the sub-bandage pressure that one expects to achieve at the ankle when a product is applied (Fig. 13.1). If these products are applied at the same levels of extension they will provide graduated compression, the pressure below the knee being less than half the pressure at the ankle.

3a 14–17 mmHg: Suitable for supporting early varicose veins. There is insufficient support to reduce oedema.

3b 18–24 mmHg: Suitable for supporting varicose veins of medium severity and mild oedema, and for preventing re-ulceration. They may be used in mixed aetiology ulceration, under medical supervision, if the ABPI is > 0.8.

Table 13.18 Bandage classification (after Thomas 1990)

Class	Bandage type	Proprietary examples
Padding	Cotton wool	Sofban™ Velband™
1	Conforming-stretch	J-fast™ Lastoetel™ Slinky™
2	Light support	Crepe BP Elastocrepe™
3a	Light compression, 14–17 mmHg	K-Crepe™ Lite press™ Elset™
3b	Moderate compression, 18–24 mmHg	Granuflex adhesive™ Veinopress™ Coban™ (cohesive) Coplus™ (cohesive)
3c	High compression, 30–40 mmHg	Setopress™ Tensopress™
3d	Extra-high compression, 50–60 mmHg	Blue line

3c 30–40 mmHg: Recommended for the treatment of venous ulceration where there is no coexisting arterial component, diabetes or vasculitis. This level of compression is also helpful for managing gross venous eczema and gross oedema provided that there is no significant heart failure.

3d 50–60 mmHg: The power of these bandages is such that they are best reserved for ankle circumferences greater than 35 cm, in the presence of severe lymphoedema.

Combinations of bandages may be applied as described in Chapter 6.

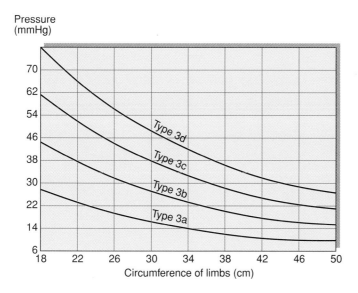

Fig. 13.1 Graph showing the relationship between the circumference of a limb and sub-bandage pressure. (After Thomas (1990))

REFERENCES

Cherry G W, Ryan T J 1985 Enhanced wound angiogenesis with a new hydrocolloid dressing. In: Ryan T J (ed) An environment for healing: the role of occlusion. International Congress and Symposium Series No. 88. Royal Society of Medicine, London

Johnson A 1988 Wound healing under the microscope. Community Outlook, January

Thomas S 1990 Bandages and bandaging; the science behind the art. Care Science and Practice 8(2)

Ting M 1991 Wound healing and peripheral vascular disease. Critical Care Nursing Clinics of North America 3(3): 515–523

FURTHER READING

Thomas S 1996 Invitro investigations of a new hydrogel dressing. Journal of Wound Care 5(3): 130–133

Thomas S, Hay N P 1994 Fluid handling properties of hydrogel dressings. Ostomy and Wound Management 41(3): 54–59

Appendices

Useful vascular abbreviations

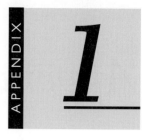

AAA	Abdominal aortic aneurysm	**LDL**	Low-density lipoproteins
ABPI	Ankle brachial pressure index	**LLLT**	Low-level laser therapy
ACE	Angiotensin-converting enzyme	**MAA**	Multi-agency assessment
ACh	Acetylcholine	**MCV**	Mean corpuscular volume
ANF	Antinuclear factor	**MCH**	Mean corpuscular haemoglobin
APTT	Activated partial thromboplastin time	**MCHC**	Mean corpuscular haemoglobin concentration
ATA	Anterior tibial artery		
BP	Blood pressure	**MHz**	Megahertz
CE	Carotid endarterectomy	**MI**	Myocardial infarction
CKMB	Creatine kinase myocardial band	**MRSA**	Methicillin-resistant *Staphylococcus aureus*
CICs	Circulating immune complexes		
CO$_2$	Carbon dioxide	**mmHg**	Millimetres of mercury
CPK	Creatine phosphokinase	**NSAID**	Non-steroidal anti-inflammatory drug
CT	Computed tomography	**PA**	Peroneal artery
CVA	Cerebrovascular accident	**Pa**	Partial pressure
CVP	Central venous pressure	**PPAM aid**	Pneumatic post-amputation mobility aid
DSA	Digital subtraction angiography	**ppm**	Parts per million
ECG	Electrocardiogram	**PTA**	Posterior tibial artery
EMA	Early mobility aid	**PTE**	Positron emission tomography
ESR	Erythrocyte sedimentation rate	**PVD**	Peripheral vascular disease
ePTFE	Expanded polytetrafluoroethylene (graft material)	**PGI$_2$**	Prostaglandin I$_2$ (prostacyclin)
		PGD$_2$	Prostaglandin D$_2$
GTN	Glyceryl trinitrate	**PGE$_1$**	Prostaglandin E$_1$
HDL	High-density lipoproteins	**rt-PA**	Tissue plasminogen activator
IPC	Intermittent pneumatic compression	**SVC**	Superior vena cava
INR	International normative ratio	**TIA**	Transient ischaemic attack
IVC	Inferior vena cava	**TXA$_2$**	Thromboxane A$_2$
LDH	Lactate dehydrogenase	**VMC**	vasomotor centre

Examples of patient information

THINGS YOU NEED TO KNOW ABOUT

COMPRESSION BANDAGES

- You have been placed in a bandage which should help any swelling in your leg to go down.
- This bandage is designed to promote healing.
- This is best achieved if you are able to leave the bandage in place until your next dressing time, which will be given to you by your nurse.
- However, if you should *ever* feel any unusual signs of discomfort, such as pins and needles, cramp, excessive coldness, blueness of the toes or a feeling that the pressure is too great, please cut off the top layer/s and leave on the bottom two layers, i.e. the cottonwool and crepe.
- Immediately phone ....
- Whilst wearing compression bandages, raise your legs as high in the air as you can whenever you sit down. They should be higher than your hips if possible.
- Do not stand still for more than a few minutes at any one time and sleep at night with your leg raised up to 45 degrees if this can be arranged safely.
- When sitting still, practise the leg exercises your nurse will show you.
- Do not sit too close to a fire, especially if cream has been applied to your leg, as this can cause blistering.
- Eat a well balanced meal. Try not to be overweight.
- Give up smoking—this will help to heal your ulcer.
- *Please ask any questions you may ever have.*

NOW THAT YOUR LEG ULCER HAS HEALED...

Now that your leg ulcer has healed … do make sure you never get another one! So …

- wear your compression stockings all day
- put them on before your feet swell—that means before you get up!
- only take them off for washing, bathing and at bedtime
- make a note of which stockings you have, so as to ask your GP for more every 3 months
  Type ....
  Size ....
  Date ....
- never get them creased or turned over at the top.
- use skin emollients, e.g. Unguentum Merck or oils such as arachis oil at night, and emollients, e.g. Oilatum or Hydromol in the bath

• ask your nurse if you need an aid to put on your stockings.

Be sure to put your stockings on first thing!

Walk everywhere if you can ...

• in comfortable shoes with a low heel
• avoid standing still
• when you have to stand, shift your weight from foot to foot and keep those ankles on the move. Even wiggle your toes.

and when you REST ...

• sit with your feet at least as high as your hips
• lie down with your feet higher than your head
• safely raise the bottom end of your bed with bricks or something solid, or blankets under the foot of the mattress
• don't wear your girdle too tightly
• don't sit with your legs crossed
• try to lose weight if you're the wrong shape.

and at MEAL TIMES ...

• eat a healthy diet: plenty of fruit & veg, chicken & fish—and lay off the fatty or sweet things. Grill, don't fry
• drink plenty of water.

Looking after your legs pays off ...

• keep them warm but not too close to the fire
• many ulcers start with an injury so take care
• don't walk barefoot
• avoid scratching
• if your legs hurt, try some mild painkillers from the chemist and talk to your nurse/doctor about it
• watch for danger signs in either leg
      pain
          swelling
             burning or other unusual sensations
                changes in colour
                    itchy, rough patches in the skin.

If you have any questions or worries, don't hesitate to contact your district nurse. The earlier things are put right, the better!

Your nurse is ....

Contact number/s ....

UNDERSTANDING CAROTID ENDARTERECTOMY

Considerations before a carotid endarterectomy

Why am I being considered for a carotid endarterectomy?

The vessels in your neck (*carotid arteries*) have become narrowed by *atheroma*. This prevents the blood from circulating freely. You may have experienced a variety of symptoms, e.g. dizziness.

Atherosclerosis is a disease process caused by the build-up in fats (cholesterol) and calcium which forms plaques of atheroma. This process hardens the arteries, which are the vessels which carry blood from the heart to the various parts of the body. The result is that the artery becomes narrowed. There is a danger that some of the atheroma might break off and travel to the brain, resulting in either mini-strokes (TIAs) or a more severe stroke (CVA).

Atherosclerosis is not a disease that you catch, but it may be that other members of your family are affected. Generally it appears in people over the age of 60, and is often associated with high blood pressure, diabetes and smoking. Stress and obesity and lack of exercise can also cause 'hardening of the arteries'.

What tests will be done?

You may have some of the tests done as an outpatient, or you may be admitted to hospital for a few days. An *ultrasound scan* (duplex) will show up any narrowing in the arteries. A clear gel is applied before an instrument which looks like a pen is run over the neck, along the line of blood vessels. The flow of blood in the vessels can then be seen. It will not hurt.

Occasionally *angiography* may be required. The radiologist injects a dye which shows up the blood vessels and any blockages on a video screen. (See angiography booklet.) The doctors will want to be certain that your general health is good. To find out they will request: blood tests, ECG (electrocardiogram shows the functioning of the heart) and a chest X-ray. The doctors will give you the results of these tests if you wish.

What happens in the operation?

The surgeon will open the vessel and scoop out the atheroma. The vessel is then closed. This may require the use of a material patch (*dacron*) to be sewn over the opening at the end of the operation. This can stay inside the body and prevents the vessel narrowing whilst being closed. You will have a wound which is approximately 12 cm/5 in long down the side of your neck. This usually heals to a fine line. If you would like to see a piece of grafting material, please do ask.

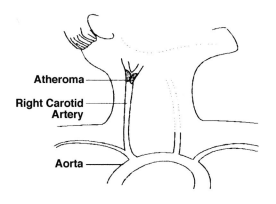

Fig. 1 Carotid arteries.

Atheroma

Right Carotid Artery

Aorta

After the operation you may find there is a *permanent numb area under your chin* due to the loss of superficial nerves, so please *take care when shaving*.

If you wish to learn more about the risks and benefits of this surgery, please discuss this with your doctor. It is important you become as *fit as possible, prior to surgery*.

How can I achieve this?

Diet If you are overweight, it is important to take a well balanced reducing diet, comprising plenty of proteins, minerals and vitamins, which will help to promote healing after your operation. It needs to contain some fat, but in small quantities, and polyunsaturated fats whenever possible. High fibre will also be beneficial in preventing constipation. Please tell the doctor/nurse if you require any special diet. A dietician is available if required by you.

Smoking Stop smoking! To reduce the risk of breathing problems, during and after your operation, it is important to stop smoking at an early stage. This will also have the added benefits of reducing the risk of further hardening of the arteries. *Nicotine patches* are now available from the chemist to help you and we will be pleased to give you advice.

Alcohol The recommended safe limit for men is 21 units and for women 14 units, spread through the week. One unit is equal to: $\frac{1}{2}$ pint of beer; 1 small glass of wine; 1 single measure of spirits.

Exercise This helps the blood to circulate around the body. It helps to keep you fit, so helping your recovery from surgery. A brisk walk each day and swimming are excellent ways of achieving this if you are able to do so. Simply rotating the feet and tightening and relaxing the calf muscles will be of some benefit, as will practising to take deep breaths.

Relaxation Stress is a factor in hardening of the arteries. High degrees of anxiety can increase stress. This can be greatly reduced through having an understanding of your situation and using relaxation techniques which the nurses will be pleased to discuss with you. If you can practise relaxing before the operation, you will be more able to do so after, so helping you to feel better more quickly. This may also help you sleep better.

Sleep Do speak with your GP if your sleep is disturbed, as it is important that you have as much proper rest as possible.

Admission to hospital for carotid endarterectomy

You may be in hospital for approximately 3–5 days, but the doctors will only send you home when they are pleased with your recovery.

You will need to bring with you soap, 2 flannels, toothbrush and toothpaste, comb/brush, shaving equipment (if used), a towel, night wear, dressing gown and slippers. A bottle of fruit juice, tissues and small change for the telephone are often useful. A Walkman radio/tape recorder is often found to aid relaxation.

The nurses will greet you and show you around the ward, informing you of the ward routine.

The house officer (doctor) will admit you to the ward and explain the operation again, as well as arranging for the above tests.

Investigations

You will be admitted to hospital the day before the operation for several tests, some of which you may have already had in clinic.

The *anaesthetist* will visit you prior to your operation and ask if you have any allergies or previous medical complaints. He may prescribe some medicine for you to take prior to the operation. You will be asked to sign a *consent* form which applies to the *operation* and the *anaesthetic*.

If necessary, the nurses may assist you to shave your neck prior to theatre. You will be told when to stop eating and drinking.

You may be given some medication to help you to sleep and relax prior to theatre.

What happens when I wake up?

For the purpose of special monitoring of your progress, it is standard practice to take all patients who have had surgery to a unit to *recover* from the *anaesthetic*, until the doctors are happy for you to return to the ward. This is usually within a few hours. Please do not worry about this. The nurses will make *routine observations* at regular intervals of your blood pressure, pulse, temperature and heart rate.

When you wake up you will find there is a *drip* in place. This is to give you clear fluids during your recovery. A blood transfusion may be required.

A *wound drainage* tube is sometimes inserted in the area of the wound's dressing. This is to remove any old blood after the operation.

How is pain and sickness controlled?

Minor discomfort is all that is usually experienced after this operation. We aim to keep you free from pain and any feeling of sickness. *Please do tell the nurses if you are uncomfortable, as there is no need for you to be so.* Pain and sickness relief drugs can be given as prescribed by the doctors, if necessary.

Oxygen via a mask or nasal tubes may be given just after your operation to aid the recovery of your breathing after having an anaesthetic.

As soon as you feel able you will be allowed to drink some water and then move on to having a light meal.

What happens over the next few days?

On the first day after the operation, the nurses will assist you to wash in bed. You may sit out for a short while. A day of rest is a wonderful tonic. Your *drip* and *wound drain* (if present) will possibly be removed. The nurses will take off the theatre dressing and may apply a clean dressing.

On the second day, you will be allowed to sit out of bed for a little longer and be able to help yourself more. By the third day, you should be feeling much more mobile. Short walks will be encouraged, until you feel strong enough to walk greater distances on the 3rd–4th day, when you may be discharged.

It is important that, while you are still in bed, you *do not cross your legs* as this restricts blood flow. *Regularly move your legs around and take deep breaths.*

Move feet up and down, rotate feet round and round.

Shaving As stated above, a patch of numbness may remain, close to the middle of the neck. It is important when shaving to be careful. Always look in the mirror to ensure you do not cut yourself.

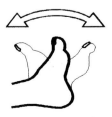 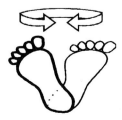

Fig. 2 Leg exercise.

The wound The skin closure is usually removed around the 5th–7th day. If the skin closures are not removed on the ward, a district nurse may be arranged to do this at home. The ward staff will make specific arrangements for you. Some numbness and itching around the wound is normal, as is some soreness as the scar tissue forms. Your scar should fade to a pale colour after 6–12 months and become less noticeable.

Life after a carotid endarterectomy

Tablets You may be given some tablets to take home with you which may include some painkillers and some antibiotics. The small dose of aspirin prescribed must be taken daily after meals, unless you are otherwise advised by a doctor. The aspirin is to help to reduce the risk of blood clots in the future as it makes the blood less sticky. You will be sent home with a small supply of drugs. Should you require any more, you should visit your GP who will have received a letter explaining what has happened during your stay in hospital. Do arrange to see the GP before the tablets run out if you need to continue with a regular dose.

Outpatients appointment When you go home, you will be given an appointment to come and see the hospital doctors in outpatients a few weeks after your discharge. This is a routine check-up after your operation.

A *check duplex* may also be arranged for this time. It is rare for further surgery to be required, but during the next 2 years you may be sent an appointment to attend the X-ray department every 6 months for a repeat scan.

When to contact your doctor/practice nurse or district nurse Do this if your wound starts to leak, looks very red or becomes extremely sore. You should also contact your doctor if you *feel generally unwell* in *any way*, e.g. *dizzy* or experiencing *headache* or *difficulty in focusing.*

Help at home If any help is needed at home, either to make your coming into hospital or your discharge easier, the nurses will be pleased to discuss this with you and help where possible.

Ongoing advice

Diet Unless there is any other underlying medical condition, there is no restriction on your diet. However, one should always bear in mind the benefits of a healthy diet.

Smoking If you have been able to stop for this operation, it is beneficial to your health not to recommence.

Alcohol Please remember the recommended daily units.

Returning to work If this is applicable, you should take 4 weeks off after your operation. If your job involves heavy lifting or is physically strenuous, you may need longer. Check with the hospital doctor before discharge or see your GP before returning.

Working at home The principle above should apply if you are retired or not working. You may feel like a sleep in the afternoon for a week or so. This is normal and to be encouraged.

Exercise Initially, during your convalescence of 2–3 weeks, a daily gentle walk in the fresh air and gentle exercise is recommended, combined with rest. Exercise such as swimming, jogging or racket sports should not be resumed for at least 4–6 weeks. Remember, the tissues and muscles inside need to heal and strengthen first. Please do check with your GP before recommencing strenuous activity.

Bathing Once your wound is dry, even before the stitches are removed, you may bath or shower.

Sexual activity You may resume your normal sex life after 2–3 weeks if you feel happy about doing so. Just be gentle at first, as you would when recommencing anything else.

Home support The ward staff will evaluate your home needs before you leave. If it is considered appropriate by you and the nursing staff, support will be arranged at home until you feel able to cope by yourself—e.g. meals on wheels, home help, etc.

In summary

Be guided by the doctors/nurses and by how you feel. Expect to be tired and weak for at least 4–6 weeks. It can take several months to fully regain your strength. This is normal. If you do have any concerns or queries, don't hesitate to contact your GP or the hospital ward and ask for advice and help.

Our best wishes go with you.

Contact name:

Booklets in this series, available from Impra UK, include: Angiogram; Angioplasty; Thrombolysis; Bypass; Aortic Aneurysm Repair; Amputation; Carotid Endarterectomy.

Useful addresses

Raynaud's Association Trust
112 Crew Road
Alsager ST7 25A
Tel: 01270 872776

National Association for Limbless
Disabled
(NALD)
31 The Mall
Ealing
London *W5*
Tel: 0181–579 1758/9

Royal Association for Disability and
Rehabilitation (RADAR)
25 Mortimer Street
London W18AB
Tel: 0171–250 3222

PACT Employment Service
Disability Services Branch
Courtwood House
Silver Street Head
Sheffield S12DD
Tel: 0114–276 8644

Banstead Mobility Centre
Damson Way
Orchard Hill
Queen Mary Avenue
Banstead SM54 MR
Tel: 0181–770 1151

Drivers' Medical Branch
DVLS
Swansea SA99 1TU
Financial benefits
(attendance allowance)
Tel: Freephone 0800–882200

Early mobility aid:
PPAM Aid
Vessa Ltd
Mill Lane
Alton GU34 2PX

Hyperbaric Oxygen Systems:
Hyox Systems Ltd
Westhill Industrial Estate
Westhill
Aberdeen AB32 6TQ

Laser therapy in wound management:
Omega Laser Systems Ltd
211 New North Rd
London N1 6UT

*Doppler ultrasound and Flotron therapy
equipment:*
Huntleigh Nesbit Evans Healthcare
310–312 Dallow Road
Luton LU1 1TD

Stocking applicator aids:
Medivallet
Fields Yard
Plough Lane
Hereford HR4 0EL

*Wound care products and compression
bandages:*
3M Health Care Products
3M House
Morley Street
Loughborough LE11 1EP

Beiersdorf
Yeomans Drive
Blakelands
Milton Keynes MK14 5LS

Convatec
Harrington House
Milton Rd
Ickenham
Uxbridge UB10 8PU

Seton
Tubiton House
Oldham OL1 3HS

Smith & Nephew
PO Box 81
Hessle Rd
Hull HU3 2BN

Impra UK
4 DeSalis Court
Hampton Lovett
Droitwich WR9 0NX

The Society of Vascular Nurses was founded by nurses for nurses. Enquiries for membership should be forwarded to:

The Membership Secretary
Vascular Nurses Society
The Vascular Unit, Level 6
John Radcliffe Infirmary
Headington
Oxford

Index